THE SCENTS OF NATURE . . .
DISTILLED INTO THE ESSENCES OF WELLNESS

DISCOVER—

- A FLORAL WATER OF GENUINE LAVENDER
TO TONE AND TIGHTEN THE SKIN (page 83)

- THE SENSUAL PLEASURE OF PATCHOULI
IN BATHWATER,
A NATURAL APHRODISIAC (page 105)

- AN OIL OF ROSE RUBBED INTO THE TEMPLES
AND NECK TO
ELEVATE MOOD AND SOOTHE A GRIEVING HEART
(page 112)

- HYSSOP DIFFUSED INTO THE AIR TO RELIEVE
THE DISCOMFORT OF **COLDS AND FLU** (page 72)

- SMOKY, WOODSY OIL OF CYPRESS TO
REDUCE SPIDER VEINS AND TREAT CELLULITE
(page 59)

- SWEET, FLOWERY YLANG-YLANG TO
RESTORE CALM
AND TURN THOUGHTS TOWARD LOVE (page 131)

THE MOST BEAUTIFUL OF THE HEALING ARTS . . .

AROMATHERAPY

The Essential Healing Arts Series:

Aromatherapy: The A–Z Guide to Healing with
   Essential Oils
Ayurveda: The A–Z Guide to Healing Techniques
   from Ancient India
Traditional Chinese Medicine: The A–Z Guide to
   Natural Healing from the Orient
Reflexology: The A–Z Guide to Healing with Pressure
   Points

AROMATHERAPY

THE A–Z GUIDE
TO HEALING
WITH ESSENTIAL OILS

SHELAGH RYAN MASLINE
AND
BARBARA CLOSE

A Lynn Sonberg Book

A Dell Book

Published by
Dell Publishing
a division of
Bantam Doubleday Dell Publishing Group, Inc.
1540 Broadway
New York, New York 10036

IMPORTANT NOTE:
Neither this nor any other book should be used as a substitute for professional medical care or treatment. It is advisable to seek the guidance of a physician or other qualified health practitioner before implementing any of the approaches to health suggested in this book. This book was written to provide selected information to the public concerning conventional and alternative medical treatments for a variety of health problems. Research in this field is ongoing and subject to interpretation. Although we have made all reasonable efforts to include the most up-to-date and accurate information in this book, there is no guarantee that what we know about this complex subject won't change with time. The reader should bear in mind that this book is not intended to take the place of medical advice from a trained medical professional. Readers are advised to consult a physician or other qualified health professional regarding treament of all of their health problems. Neither the publisher, the producer, nor the authors take any responsibility for any possible consequences from any treatment, action, or application of medicine or preparation by any person reading or following the information in this book.

ISBN: 0-440-22256-7

Published by arrangement with: Lynn Sonberg Book Associates, 260 West 72 Street, New York, N.Y. 10023

Printed in the United States of America

Published simultaneously in Canada

January 1998

10 9 8 7 6 5 4 3 2

OPM

This book is dedicated with great love and affection
to my daughter
Caitlin Ryan,
and to my mother
Eileen Ryan.

CONTENTS

FOREWORD

The rapid growth of the aromatherapy industry is part of an increasing interest in natural health and complementary medicine as a whole. Suddenly how we view conventional medicine is being questioned not only within the health care establishment as it seeks to cut costs but also by consumers themselves, who feel frustrated by the options available to them. In particular, individuals suffering from chronic conditions—illnesses that develop gradually over a period of time and have no clearly defined remedy—are seeking new ways to heal themselves. As a result we have seen a growing interest in alternative healing arts such as aromatherapy, herbal medicine, acupuncture, and homeopathy—not to replace Western medicine but to serve as a useful ally in healing.

This book is a concise, comprehensive, and accessible guide for newcomers to the field of aromatherapy. It provides an overview of the benefits of aromatherapy in enhancing our pleasure, health, and well-being. Many people believe that aromatherapy is not truly a healing art. On the contrary a wealth of scientific literature validating the psychological and physiological benefits of essential oils is being published nowadays in England, France, Germany, and Japan. In England essential oils have been introduced in hospitals to address a number of health problems, and their benefits have been documented in powerful case studies. In France and Germany essential oils are often prescribed by physicians to treat any number of health conditions. Several large corporations in Japan have utilized essential oils for their psychological benefits in increasing workers' productivity and performance. These exciting developments help weave the delicate path between art and science and should, in the years to come, change how people in the United States view aromatherapy, enabling them to see it as something more than a fashionable trend.

At my healing-arts center in New York I have witnessed firsthand the miracles of essential oils in addressing a number of health problems, from digestive complaints to skin disorders to a range of stress-related illnesses. Clients are not only excited to see their conditions improve but also learn to care for themselves without the cost and unpleasant side effects of more aggressive drugs.

Whether you are a newcomer to the art and science of aromatherapy or have been enjoying the benefits of essential oils for years, this book will give you much to intrigue and inspire the senses and promote a better sense of well-being. Enjoy!

Barbara Close
B.C. Botanicus, October 1996

HOW TO USE THIS BOOK

In *Aromatherapy: The A–Z Guide to Healing with Essential Oils,* you will have an opportunity to learn about the many ways that aromatherapy can safely and effectively ease your health and beauty concerns. Chapter 1 provides you with a sound introduction to how aromatherapy works and a brief history of the ways in which essential oils have been used through the ages. You will also see how modern scientific applications of aromatherapy were born in twentieth-century France.

Chapter 2 explains how we put theory into practice. There are many ways to use essential oils, and you can read all about them in this chapter. This chapter underscores the need to recognize and avoid synthetic essential oils, which are frequently used in the fragrance industry but lack the therapeutic benefits of natural essential oils. In addition care has been taken to emphasize the invaluable aid of the carrier oils with which essential oils are mixed.

Turn to Chapter 3 to find detailed profiles of more than fifty of the most commonly used essential oils, including their functions in health and beauty and any safety precautions you should take while using them. Each essential oil possesses its own unique set of characteristics. For example some are stimulating while others are calming; certain oils act as fitting complements to the medical care of bronchitis or flu, while others are just the thing for relieving sore muscles in a postworkout massage. Essential oils are organized in alphabetical order for easy reference.

In Chapter 4 you can look up your own personal health and beauty concerns and learn about supportive aromatherapy for them. A variety of treatments are suggested for each symptom or condition so that you can mix and match to find the recipe that is right for you. As in Chapter 3, entries are arranged in alphabetical order for ease of use. From acne to constipation, hair care to hangovers, jet lag to stress to sexuality to wounds—in this section you will find a variety of easy-to-prepare remedies using therapeutic essential oils.

Essential oils are growing in popularity and are becoming more and more accessible at your local health food store. But just in case they haven't yet made their way to your town, the book closes with a source list of reputable mail-order suppliers of high-quality essential oils.

CHAPTER ONE

THE ART OF AROMATHERAPY

Aromatherapy is the art of using essential oils from plants and trees to protect and enhance your health, beauty, and overall well-being. When modern medicine was developed earlier this century, we temporarily lost sight of aromatherapy, along with many other natural approaches to our wellness. Yet the 1990s have witnessed an overwhelming renaissance of interest in alternative treatments. And, with effects that range from relaxation to stimulation, you may find aromatherapy to be the safe and natural answer to many of your own health and beauty concerns.

WHAT IS AROMATHERAPY?

Essential oils, which are distilled from plants, flowers, trees, fruits, and herbs, have been prized since ancient times for their impact on both the body and the mind.

These substances possess a virtual medicine cabinet full of healing abilities; their effects range from analgesic to antidepressant to antiseptic to anti-inflammatory to antibiotic to antiviral. Essential oils can have a definite impact on your emotional state, and are used to treat a wide range of physical ills as well.

Aromatherapy has a wide variety of applications, and to accomplish your desired effect—whether that may be to relieve stress, alleviate headache pain, soothe a stomachache, or rehydrate aging dry skin—you may diffuse essential oils into the air you breathe, create body oils for massage, or add a few drops to a bath, compress, cosmetic lotion, or hydrolat (a floral water in spritzer or spray form). In this chapter you will learn all about the theory behind aromatherapy.

ESSENTIAL OILS ARE FOR EXTERNAL USE

The two most effective ways to use essential oils are inhalation and external application in baths or preparations such as massage oils. In Europe essential oils are also sometimes recommended for internal use, but this is not common in our country. In the United States we take a more cautious approach to alternative remedies; while scientific evidence supports the safe and effective use of therapeutic essential oils on an external basis, the jury is still out on their internal use. An inappropriate internal use of essential oils could result in a variety of ill effects, ranging from a simple case of indigestion to a serious toxic reaction. This is why we recommend essential oils *for external use only.*

AROMATHERAPY AND CONVENTIONAL MEDICINE

Aromatherapy is a safe and natural way to help keep you healthy in mind and body. However, it is *not* intended to be a replacement for conventional medicine. Nor is it meant to be the sole treatment for any critical illness. In case of any serious medical problem it is possible that aromatherapy can *complement* your regular treatment by easing discomfort and relieving anxiety. You can feel safe and secure in the knowledge that aromatherapy can peacefully coexist with your normal medical care.

Chances are that not only will your doctor not object to a whiff of peppermint to counteract your motion sickness (a common practice in aromatherapy), she may applaud your resourcefulness in finding a natural alternative to medications for motion sickness, which often have unwanted and unnecessary side effects. Likewise a massage with the musky scent of patchouli may be just the thing to spice up your love life, and is not likely to set off any medical alarms. You can also use aromatherapy—and other techniques such as meditation, music, and yoga—side by side with traditional medicine to help relieve tension and stress that may lead to potentially serious health problems, such as depression, headache, and high blood pressure.

A NEW FREEDOM FROM SIDE EFFECTS

For day-to-day aches and pains aromatherapy can provide a natural and side-effect-free alternative to the bottles lining your medicine cabinet. Many women turn to aromatherapy because they'd rather try a soothing lavender or vanilla bath than a pill to relieve headache pain. And after a stressful day at the office a relaxing massage with your favorite essential oil can replace a tranquilizer, leaving your mind more alert to cope with preparing dinner or picking up your daughter from tennis practice.

The fact is we are much more aware of the side effects of the drugs we take today—that is, of their potential impact on both our bodies and minds. Regular use of common over-the-counter remedies such as aspirin and ibuprofen has been linked to gastrointestinal disturbances, while prescription drugs such as tranquilizers are potentially addictive and can leave you feeling groggy and disoriented instead of revitalized and refreshed. Essential oils, on the other hand, are usually excreted from the body within three to six hours and leave no toxins behind.

Why not try the natural way first? In fact if you suffer from common ailments such as borderline high blood pressure, excess weight, or cholesterol that is edging up over the 200 level, most doctors today encourage you to try to get a grip on your health through diet, exercise, and stress reduction. There is virtually universal agreement that medications should be prescribed only when health problems are serious and natural measures are insufficient to control them. A number of health maintenance organizations, or HMOs, are even cautiously joining in this trend; reimbursements are on the rise for patients who participate in programs that emphasize preventive health and the mind-body connection.

THE THREE TYPES OF AROMATHERAPY

Aromatherapy is sometimes mistakenly thought to be related to beauty issues only. Botanical shampoos and moisturizers are extremely popular today, and well-known commercial hair treatments such as VO5 now advertise that they include essential oils in their mix.

These practices are part of what we call aesthetic aromatherapy, and there is no question that the wider availability of natural products—especially those incorporating essential oils—is a great addition to regular skin and hair care. But in fact aromatherapy can also be used therapeutically to help heal common physical ailments as well as psychological ills.

When your mind is at peace, your body is less likely to plague you with nervous stomachaches and headaches. Even more important you need to control stress and tension, since they have been linked to a weakening of the immune system and potentially dangerous health conditions such as high blood pressure. As for healthy skin and hair, they come from the inside out. With proper diet, regular exercise, and freedom from undue levels of stress, your skin will enjoy more life and color and less susceptibility to troublesome rashes.

So while there is a great deal of overlap, we can generally group the practice of aromatherapy into three areas:

- **Psychoaromatherapy** is the use of essential oils to help resolve emotional imbalances and enhance psychological wellness and harmony. Through inhalation or the external application of essential oils in massages or baths, the brain may be either relaxed or stimulated. Grounding essential oils such as sandalwood and frankincense have a calming and tranquilizing effect, inducing a general sense of well-being; they relieve the restless and agitated mind and are especially helpful in the relief of stress and anxiety. Stimulating oils such as rosemary and cardamom are energizing; they can help pull you out of a funk, relieving depression and general malaise.

- **Aesthetic Aromatherapy** refers to the inclusion of essential oils in your beauty routine. The use of therapeutic essential oils can easily become a regular part of your skin and hair care. Some essential oils can be used to regulate the production of sebum, an oily substance that keeps your skin smooth and moist. Overproduction of sebum—a common problem in adolescence—can lead to acne; as we grow older, sebum production slows, resulting in dry skin. Other essential oils stimulate circulation and encourage the growth of new skin. Many oils can be applied to remoisturize, rehydrate, and rejuvenate aging skin. If you're a brunette, rosemary oil can help keep your hair shiny and clean, while blondes can benefit from the addition of a little German chamomile to their shampoo.

- **Therapeutic Aromatherapy** harnesses the natural analgesic, antiseptic, anti-inflammatory, antibiotic, and antiviral qualities of essential oils for healing purposes. For example lavender, which contains a high concentration of naturally antiseptic linalol, can be spritzed on the skin during long flights, when stale air is constantly recirculated. A soothing rosemary massage can relieve sore muscles by increasing local circulation and helping to remove lactic acid and cellular waste products.

How Essential Oils Work

Essential oils are highly concentrated extracts of plants containing a wide variety of complex chemical compounds. When you inhale their scents, you stimulate the olfactory nerve endings at the bridge of your nose. From here the fragrances of essential oils are sent directly to the limbic portion of your brain, where the impact of their chemical components is immediate and dramatic.

The limbic system is the home of our autonomic nervous system, which is responsible for our sexuality, our likes and dislikes, our moods and impulses, our creativity. At the root of the cerebral cortex, the limbic system belongs to one of the earliest and most primitive regions of the brain, making the sense of smell one of our most primal and fundamental senses.

When scents reach the limbic system, the brain responds by releasing its own natural relaxants or stimulants, which are chemicals called neurotransmitters. Neurotransmitters include endorphins, serotonin, and noradrenaline. Endorphins are natural painkillers, relaxants, and increase our sense of pleasure; serotonin is calming and helps regulate appetite; noradrenaline is stimulating. Tranquilizing essential oils include jasmine, orange, and rose; stimulating oils are rosemary, basil, and cardamom.

Through their impact on the limbic system of the brain, scents influence our emotions and psychological functions. Research has shown that oils such as jasmine, orange, and rose alter brain waves into a calm pattern, while oils including basil and rosemary are naturally stimulating.

AROMAS UNLOCK OUR MEMORIES

Scents also evoke powerful memories, and memories of aromas are stored in the limbic system. You can harness these scents and reawaken these "comfort" memories, in much the same way that people turn to the "comfort" foods of childhood for occasional solace. And keep in mind that scent memories are far less fattening than mashed potatoes, chocolate, and other classic comfort foods!

When I smell vanilla, I am brought back to sunny afternoons in the kitchen baking chocolate bits with my mother and aunt. The smell of pine is forever associated with the snowy Christmas mornings of childhood. Many of us associate the scent of lavender with our mothers or grandmothers, women of another generation, and perhaps memories of them—in addition to the fact that lavender contains soothing chemical components known as esters—is one of the reasons that lavender is such a universally loved fragrance.

THE HISTORY OF AROMATHERAPY

Our ancestors long ago experimented with plants, gradually identifying by trial and error those that were nutritious, those with healing abilities, and others that were poisonous and to be avoided. If you have a dog or cat, you will probably see your pet doing the same thing today. Veterinarians believe that many animals deliberately consume grass to make them vomit, a natural way of cleansing their bodies of toxins.

Looking back through history, we can see that aromatic substances have been used since ancient times for health and for worship. Famous physicians of history, such as the Greek Hippocrates and the Arab Avicenna, prescribed aromatic oils to their patients to cure disease. Greek and Roman bath houses were scented with aromatic oils to promote relaxation and hygiene. According to Hippocrates, the road to good health was paved with a daily aromatic bath and massage. That advice continues to be true today.

The ancient Greeks also burned aromatic substances in the streets to prevent the spread of contagious disease, and a legacy of this practice continues to exist in European hospitals today, where naturally antiseptic lavender is still used to purify and disinfect the air. The Greeks considered essential oils to be a gift from the gods, and perhaps they are.

The Perfumes of Ancient Egypt

In ancient Egypt substances resembling the essential oils we use today were applied as both medicines and perfumes. Perfumes containing angelica, cedarwood, juniper, and myrrh were burned like incense to perfume the air. Legend has it that Cleopatra wore the sensual fragrance of jasmine to bring Mark Antony around to her point of view.

The ancient Egyptians knew even then that certain aromas were stimulating and could increase the powers of concentration, while others induced tranquillity. Essential oils were sacred substances used to embalm Egyptian pharaohs. When King Tut's tomb was unearthed earlier this century, traces of frankincense and myrrh were among the many treasures detected.

Aromatherapy Arrives in the Twentieth Century

Although the practice of aromatherapy stretches back to Antony and Cleopatra, the term itself was coined by the French scientist René-Maurice Gattefossé in 1938. Dr. Gattefossé accidentally discovered the healing properties of lavender when he severely burned himself in a laboratory experiment. He immediately immersed his throbbing hand in a nearby bowl of liquid, which happened to be pure lavender oil. Not only was the pain relieved but the burn quickly healed.

The use of essential oils has become increasingly

widespread since Dr. Gattefossé's fortuitous accident. In Europe alternative approaches such as aromatherapy and herbalism never fell into the disregard they suffered in the United States, and research into them has continued virtually unabated.

In Japan researchers at Shinsen (the third largest cosmetics company in the world) discovered that giving women facials scented with orange and tangerine lowered their blood pressure. In Tokyo large corporations circulate the aromas of lemon and peppermint through the air-conditioning to help increase workers' concentration and focus.

Aromatherapy and You

In our own country aromatherapy is also beginning to experience something of an official welcome. Hospitals such as Memorial Sloan-Kettering in New York City are using essential oils to relax patients during MRIs (magnetic resonance imagings). Your own introduction to aromatherapy can be as close as your neighborhood health food store.

Whether you want to reduce the use of medicines that may have unpleasant side effects, assume greater control over your own health, or simply try a new and intriguing way of addressing your health and cosmetic concerns, you may want to give safe and natural aromatherapy a try.

Wherever your motivation stems from, you will learn in this book that aromatherapy is a gentle yet effective way you can take advantage of your innate healing powers and move a few steps closer to your personal wellness and beauty goals. Aromatherapy is especially suited to self-care and, like a balanced diet and regular exercise, can easily be incorporated into your healthy lifestyle. Read on to learn more about how essential oils can work for you.

CHAPTER TWO

A PRACTICAL GUIDE TO ESSENTIAL OILS

In this chapter you will learn more practical information about how to buy and apply essential oils. We know now that there are two primary ways we can harness the healing powers of essential oils: inhalation and external application. Here we will look more closely at the specific hands-on methods whereby you can incorporate essential oils into your day-to-day health and beauty routines. At the close of this chapter you will also learn basic safety measures to keep in mind when using any remedy.

HOW ESSENTIAL OILS ARE MADE

An enormous amount of time, energy, and expertise are necessary to produce a very small amount of essential oil. For example it takes thirty pounds of leaves to produce one pound of lavender oil; one thousand pounds of blossoms for one pound of jasmine oil; and two thousand pounds of petals for one pound of rose oil!

Very strict conditions are often necessary to obtain the best essential oils. Sandalwood trees must be thirty years old before their wood is sufficiently mature to yield essential oil, while jasmine blossoms must be gathered before sunrise, when their delicate fragrance begins to evaporate.

Most essential oils are produced by steam distillation from flowers, plants, and trees. Plants are natural chemical factories, and an average essential oil may contain as many as a hundred different components, such as alcohols, esters, phenols, ketones, and terpenes. These compounds, which are up to one hundred times more concentrated than dried herbs, work on many levels. Other complex production methods—such as cold pressing, enfleurage, and maceration—are also used to make essential oils.

The best essential oils are made from natural—preferably organic—sources. Synthetic or adulterated oils cannot duplicate the therapeutic abilities of these pure extracts of plants, trees, and flowers.

Buying Essential Oils

The finest essential oils are natural, organic essential oils, which are often distilled at small, family-owned farms. Aromatherapists call these vintage essential oils, since they know and can trust their source. Just like fine wines, these essential oils vary from year to year according to climate, soil conditions, and the care taken in their cultivation. With essential oils as with wines, certain vineyards produce superior products year after year.

Not surprisingly pure essential oils can be very expensive. The price of a small bottle of essential oil can easily range from a few dollars to a few hundred dollars. Since a small amount of essential oil lasts a very long time, it is always better to purchase the real thing from a reputable source, even if the price seems a little steep.

Synthetic chemical copies of essential oils are commonly available for lower prices, as are adulterated versions, which combine a tiny amount of the real essential oil with a large quantity of a less expensive, less pure, and less effective essential oil. If essential oils are not obtained from organic sources, they may have been treated with pesticides; impurities may call their effectiveness into question.

Chemical "impostors" are not likely to have the same therapeutic effect as high-quality essential oils, and in some cases have even been known to cause rashes and other allergic reactions. What looks like an inexpensive bargain is likely to be a synthetic version made from chemicals or an adulterated version diluted with inexpensive and less effective essential oils. In either case you will receive little therapeutic value from your so-called bargain.

In most metropolitan areas essential oils are as close as your local health food store. Because oils may vary in quality, it is important to buy them from a reputable store or manufacturer so that you know you are getting the real thing. This is particularly true because there is little information on the label to help you distinguish the real thing from the impostor. Since essential oils are not available in all corners of the United States, you may find yourself at a loss when you try to find a certain remedy. Fortunately many manufacturers offer essential oils by mail. If you're still not sure which essential oil is right for you, many companies even offer starter kits of the most useful and popular ones.

Write, call, or fax the companies listed at the close of

this book for a current catalog or brochure. Often valuable informational material about current trends in aromatherapy is available as well. Many manufacturers stock hard-to-find books on aromatherapy; price lists are usually enclosed. The renowned Pacific Institute of Aromatherapy also offers correspondence courses and seminars around the country on aromatherapy.

HOW TO STORE ESSENTIAL OILS

Essential oils should be kept in tightly closed glass bottles in a cool place away from bright light. Brown bottles are best, and a medicine cabinet or the shelf of a closet will do for a safe storage location.

Some oils—especially citrus oils such as lemon, grapefruit, and orange—evaporate quickly. Be extra sure to keep their bottles tightly closed and away from sunlight. Citrus oils should remain clear; any cloudiness may indicate spoilage that can lead to skin problems. Other essential oils, like fine wines, actually improve with age. These include clary sage, patchouli, sandalwood, and vetiver.

DILUTE ESSENTIAL OILS WITH CARRIER OILS BEFORE USE

Essential oils are volatile substances that evaporate quickly upon exposure to the air. They are also highly concentrated powerful substances, and for both these reasons they are rarely used undiluted. In the vast majority of cases essential oils are blended with carrier or base oils, such as sweet almond, arnica, grapeseed, jojoba, or wheat germ. Carrier oils often have therapeutic properties themselves. This is especially true of herbal-infused carrier oils such as arnica (an excellent remedy for aches and pains) and calendula (which is helpful in the healing of wounds). In most cases you can choose your own carrier oil; in cases when certain oils are better than others, we recommend them in Chapter 4 under each health and beauty concern.

Throughout this book you will find references to carrier or vegetable carrier oils and the number of drops of an essential oil to be diluted with a given amount of a base or carrier oil. Although quantities vary, the ratio is usually three to five drops of an essential oil to one tablespoon of a carrier oil. Again, these ratios are clearly spelled out under each health and beauty concern in Chapter 4.

Most carrier oils are made from vegetables, nuts, or seeds. For the sake of purity, carrier oils should be cold pressed. This means that, in contrast to the vegetable oils found on your supermarket shelves, you can be more certain of their freedom from chemical additives and pesticides. Some carrier oils—such as arnica, calendula, evening primrose, and St. John's wort—are made from herbs. Good-quality carrier oils are generally available from the same sources as essential oils—that is, a local health food store you trust or one of the mail-order sources we recommend at the end of this book.

Essential oils also mix readily with alcohol and water. Rose and lavender water are favorites for beauty concerns, but whenever you use water, remember to shake the mixture before each use. It's important to keep in mind that most essential oils alone are too powerful to use directly on skin and may cause rashes or other difficulties if misused. In the rare instances when essential oils can be applied neat or undiluted, we state this under the profile of the essential oil in Chapter 3 and under its various applications in Chapter 4.

CARRIER OILS IN AROMATHERAPY

Essential oils are usually mixed with carrier oils, which have "fixative" qualities that balance and stabilize essential oils in massage oils, compresses, poultices, and other preparations. The following carrier oils are available from your neighborhood health food store or from the mail-order sources listed at the close of this book:

Sweet Almond—Rich in protein, helps relieve dryness and inflammation.

Apricot Kernel—Light in texture, excellent for facial massage, good for all skin problems.

Arnica—An herbal-infused oil excellent for bruises, aches, strains, and joint inflammation. Arnica should never be used on broken skin.

Avocado—Penetrating oil rich in vitamins A, B, and C.

Borage—A nutritive skin oil, high in essential fatty acids.

Calendula—An herbal-infused oil healing to wounds of all kinds, invaluable for the treatment of skin diseases.

Camellia—A light Japanese emollient for hair.

Devil's Claw—An antirheumatic herbal-infused oil good for stiff joints.

Evening Primrose—An herbal-infused oil high in gamma linolenic acid, excellent for women's health concerns, heart disease, and skin problems.

Grapeseed—Good for all skin types.

Hazelnut—Slightly astringent, good for oily or combination skin.

Jojoba—Structurally similar to skin and highly penetrating, excellent for hair care and skin problems.

Lime Blossom—An herbal-infused oil that is soothing to skin.

Rose Hip—Excellent for mature skin.

Safflower—Good for all skin types.

St. John's Wort—An herbal-infused oil with immune-enhancing, antiviral, and anti-inflammatory properties. Good for bruises, minor burns (including sunburn), psoriasis, varicose veins, and wounds.

Sesame—Rich in vitamins and minerals, good for all skin types.

Soya Bean—Good for all skin types.

Squalene—Structurally similar to sebum, derived from olives.

Sunflower—Good for all skin types.

Wheat Germ—Good for prematurely aged skin, wheat germ acts as a preservative due to its high vitamin E content. This is good to add to any mixture to keep it from turning.

A VARIETY OF ESSENTIAL-OIL PREPARATIONS

Essential oils can be inhaled or absorbed through the skin using external applications. These potent aromatic substances may be added to a warm bath, massaged into the skin, or included in a variety of other preparations including hydrolats, compresses, clay masks, lotions, and creams. Here we define the various methods of using essential oils in clear, straightforward language. Read on to learn of the many ways in which you can enjoy and employ the fragrances of aromatherapy.

INHALING ESSENTIAL OILS

Essential oils can be inhaled in any number of ways. Try adding them to your bath, to your environment via an aroma lamp or ring, or tuck a handkerchief with a drop of your favorite essential oil into a pocket or handbag.

Other ways to circulate the fragrances of essential oils include

- A drop in a nearby bowl of warm water.
- A drop in the humidifier or on the radiator.
- A drop diluted in a cup of water and thrown on the rocks in a sauna.
- A drop on a cool light bulb before switching on a lamp. (Do *not* place on a hot light bulb; you may cause it to burst.)
- A drop in the melted wax surrounding a lit candle. (Do *not* place directly on the lit wick.)

Fragrant Care for Your Air

Aroma lamps and rings—which can be made of clay, glass, or metal—are specially designed to heat essential oils so that their molecules can be diffused into the air around you. Most essential oils are naturally antiseptic, making them excellent room fresheners and germ killers during flu season. Certain scents, such as patchouli and sandalwood, are lush and sensual, while orange is a cheerful aroma to circulate for a child's birthday party.

Make Your Bath a Transcendent Experience

A luxurious therapeutic bath is one of the most sensuous and enjoyable ways to inhale essential oils; an additional benefit is that essential oils in the bath are also absorbed through the skin. Shape your bath to suit your purpose: Bring a book to read in the bathtub, or take a leisurely bath by candlelight. An inflatable bath pillow adds to your ability to relax. Take a bath to soothe tired muscles, calm frazzled nerves, meditate, or fight off a cold. A lukewarm bath for twenty minutes is a good choice; hotter and longer baths can be very drying to the skin.

To create your aromatic bath, dilute three to five drops of your favorite essential oil with a tablespoon of carrier oil and add to still bath water. Swish the water around to disperse molecules. Do not add essential oils to baths while the water is running; essential oils are so volatile that they will evaporate before you get a full chance to enjoy their therapeutic effect.

External Application of Essential Oils

Massages, baths, hydrolats, creams, lotions, and compresses are all terrific external methods to capture the healing powers of essential oils. Essential oils, because of their small molecular structure and also because they are lipid (fat) soluble, are very easily absorbed through the skin. As they penetrate the epidermis, or outer layer of skin, oils are absorbed by the small capillaries of the underlying dermis, entering the bloodstream and lymph system in about twenty minutes and circulating throughout the body.

Healing Massage

Massage seems to do it all. One of the best ways to maintain muscle tone and release muscle tension is through massage. You can also massage sore muscles to increase blood and lymph circulation and remove toxins such as lactic acid and cellular waste products. Massage induces relaxation and emotional well-being, and all these effects combine to strengthen your resistance to disease.

To prepare a massage oil, dilute three to five drops of an essential oil with a tablespoon of a carrier oil. You can massage most body parts, including the back, stomach, legs, feet, hands, face, temples, and neck.

Pamper Your Feet

Soothe your tired, aching feet with a five- to fifteen-minute soak in a bowl of warm water accented with three to five drops of an essential oil. Whether you spend your day chasing toddlers or trading stocks, your feet will benefit from this little bit of extra loving care. And if you happen to be a runner or a dancer, proper foot care and hygiene is even more important. Juniper, cypress, peppermint, rosemary, and tea tree are all good choices for foot baths. If you suffer from foot odor, keep in mind that cypress and tea tree are natural deodorants.

A New Tradition: The European Sitzbath

Sitzbaths are a traditional European remedy that have only recently become popular in this country. A sitzbath is a bath in which you immerse your pelvis in water. One of the first times a woman may hear of a sitzbath is after giving birth, if she has had an episiotomy or tear in the perineum. A sitzbath with astringent cypress and soothing lavender will encourage healing of the perineum.

You can take a sitzbath in a small bowl or shallow tub. Sitzbaths can also be used to treat hemorrhoids, menstrual problems, urinary tract problems, and yeast infections. A warm soak for ten to fifteen minutes a day is usually sufficient. Lavender, tea tree, and yarrow are among the most suitable essential oils for sitzbaths.

Treat Yourself to a Facial Steambath

A facial steambath opens your pores for deep cleansing, and its stimulation gives your skin a rosy glow. You can make your own steambath by adding three to five drops of an essential oil to a quart of hot water. Cover your head with a towel and enjoy.

Spritz Yourself with Your Favorite Hydrolat

One of the best ways to maintain clear, healthy skin is to spray your face regularly with hydrolats (floral waters). Lavender and rosewater are favorites, and lavender is especially useful since it is good for all skin types, from normal to dry to oily.

Try a Clay Mask On for Size

Face masks are made from green, red, yellow, white, black, and brown clays to treat a variety of skin conditions. Face masks can help control the overactive skin that leads to acne, rehydrate dry skin, or stimulate and rejuvenate aging skin.

Green is the finest clay, since the clay itself is balancing and revitalizing. Then, as needed, you may add a drop of geranium to tone normal skin, rosemary for oily skin, or chamomile for dry skin.

If you don't care for masks, essential oils can also be added to cosmetic creams and lotions, hand and body lotions, and face creams.

SAFETY GUIDELINES WHEN USING ESSENTIAL OILS

As we have seen, aromatherapy is a safe and natural way to maintain and enhance the wellness of both body and mind. Yet it's important to keep in mind that each essential oil is made up of a highly concentrated combination of active chemical constituents, and certain basic precautions should be taken when using aromatherapy.

The profile of every essential oil in this book concludes with a section on precautions. In general it's important to practice good old-fashioned common sense with essential oils, just as you would with any other remedy. Here are a few simple safety tips to keep in mind when using essential oils:

- Essential oils should almost always be diluted before use. The exceptions (such as lavender on an insect bite) are clearly spelled out. Otherwise carefully follow the formulas for combining essential oils with carrier or base oils.

- It's important to perform a skin test before using any diluted essential oil. This is especially true if you are prone to allergies or if you are using essential oils to treat a child or an elderly person. Put one drop of diluted essential oil on a cotton swab and with it lightly touch the inside of the elbow or back of the wrist. Leave the area unwashed. If there is no reaction after twenty-four hours, the oil is safe to use. If there is any redness or irritation, wait a day or two and test an alternative essential oil.

- Always wash your hands after using essential oils, and avoid getting oil into your eyes or other sensitive body areas.

- If you are pregnant or nursing a child, be sure to consult your obstetrician or midwife before using essential oils. Certain essential oils (such as rosemary) should be avoided during pregnancy; this information is included in the "Precautions" section of the profile of every essential oil.

- Most essential oils should be used with caution in children under two. There are of course exceptions to this guideline. A warm chamomile poultice on baby's tummy when she is suffering from colic is a safe and often effective remedy.

- If you are over sixty-five, suffer from a chronic or serious illness, or take prescription or over-the-counter medications on a regular basis, you should consult your medical professional to make certain that essential oils are safe for you to use.

- Essential oils are combustible. Do not put them on a hot light bulb or on the lit wick of a candle. (You may place a drop on a cool light bulb before turning on the switch, or in the melted wax surrounding a lit candle.)

- *Essential oils are for external use only!* The internal use of essential oils is not recommended or covered in this book.

*

CHAPTER THREE

THE A–Z GUIDE TO OVER 50 ESSENTIAL OILS

In this chapter you will find profiles of more than fifty of the most commonly used essential oils. For easy use and accessibility this chapter is organized alphabetically according to the common name of each essential oil.

By now you know that the best essential oils are those that are made naturally and organically, preferably from known producers. Sometimes, because so much work goes into the production of very small amounts of essential oil, prices may seem steep. Fortunately a very small amount of an essential oil yields great therapeutic value and one tiny bottle of essential oil will last for a very long time. There is no replacement for authenticity; synthetic or otherwise adulterated oils cannot have the same therapeutic values as pure oils.

You will also see once more in this chapter that highly concentrated essential oils are almost always combined with carrier or base oil before use. While the quantities of essential oil to carrier oil will vary, you should generally use three to five drops of essential oil to one tablespoon of carrier oil.

In a few cases essential oils can be applied neat, or undiluted. For example a drop of lavender or tea tree can be placed directly on a cut or scrape. In other cases very potent essential oils should be used in much smaller ratios to carrier oils. You will find this information clearly spelled out in each individual profile in this chapter, as well as under individual health and beauty concerns in Chapter 4.

Essential oils are safe, natural, and healthy additions to your lifestyle. Yet it is always important to pay close attention to the precautions you should take when using any remedy, and specific precautions are detailed at the close of each profile. Under precautions you will learn which oils—such as cinnamon and clove—are most likely to cause skin irritation and should be used with the greatest care. (Turn back to the close of Chapter 2 for a more extensive discussion of safety tips when using essential oils.)

Each essential profile in this chapter includes:

- The common and botanical names of the essential oil
- Its general description
- Parts of the plant or tree used to produce the oil
- The functions of the essential oil in health and in beauty
- Any precautions you should take while using this essential oil

ANGELICA

(*Angelica archangelica*)

Angelica is a European plant that has been used for healing purposes since medieval times. Legend has it that the Archangel Raphael brought angelica to a monk during the plague, when it was taken internally by caregivers to prevent infection and burned like incense to purify the air.

Today the essential oil of angelica continues to have a wide variety of uses in aromatherapy. Angelica is strengthening and rejuvenating, and inhaling its essential oil is said to reduce anxiety, stimulate the immune system, and increase energy and circulation. Try mixing angelica with eucalyptus in an aroma lamp to prevent the spread of colds and viruses during flu season. Angelica combines well with bergamot, clary sage, eucalyptus, juniper, lemongrass, pine, and tea tree.

PARTS USED: Roots and seeds

FOR HEALTH:

- The essential oil of angelica may be circulated through the air via an aroma lamp, ring, or diffuser to combat stress and anxiety.

- Angelica can also be used in this way to treat nausea and weakness during convalescence and chronic disease.

- Angelica may be dispersed into the environment to prevent the spread of germs.

- Angelica is often inhaled to improve lung and sinus congestion due to colds, coughs, flu, and sinus infections.

- To speed the healing of bruises and scars, apply a cool compress made with several drops of angelica diluted with a tablespoon of vegetable carrier oil. Use up to three times daily.

- A massage oil containing angelica may help relieve stomach cramps, PMS, menstrual discomfort, menopausal symptoms, and arthritic pain.

FOR BEAUTY:

- Angelica may be used in perfumes. In fact it was distilled into one of the world's early perfumes, Carmelite water, in the Middle Ages.

PRECAUTIONS:

Angelica is generally a safe and effective essential oil. However, when applied topically to your skin, be careful about exposure to the sun. Exposure to sunlight or ultraviolet light after use may cause a skin rash.

BASIL

(*Ocimum basilicum*)

Basil is a powerful and pungent stimulating oil used to relieve nervousness and fatigue. At times in its long history basil has been considered an aphrodisiac and a symbol of fertility. French aromatherapists in this century have noted the regulating effect of basil oil on the menstrual cycle, as well as its antitoxic properties when used to treat bites and stings. Basil combines well with other essential oils, such as grapefruit and lime.

PARTS USED: Flowers and leaves

FOR HEALTH:

- Combine a drop of basil oil with a tablespoon of vegetable carrier oil and massage over the body for an invigorating wake-me-up.

- Inhale basil to improve your concentration.

- The restorative qualities of basil oil may help regulate menstruation. If you experience PMS, try rubbing a massage oil containing basil in circles around the stomach area.

- Basil oil may also be a helpful remedy during menopause. As in the case of PMS, massage the abdomen with the diluted oil, or add a drop of basil oil to your bath.

- A cool basil compress may be applied to lessen the itching and stinging of insect bites or bee stings.

- A drop of basil oil diluted with a tablespoon of vegetable carrier oil may be gently rubbed into the temples to soothe headache pain.

- For bad breath, add a drop of basil oil to a cup of water and use as a mouthwash.

PRECAUTIONS:

Because basil oil is thought to affect the menstrual cycle, it should not be used during pregnancy. Basil is otherwise a safe and effective essential oil.

BAY

(*Pimenta acris*)

The essential oil of bay, which comes mainly from the Virgin Islands, has a strong, spicy aroma reminiscent of clove. Like clove, bay contains the chemical eugenol, which has natural antiseptic and analgesic qualities.

Bay has a long history of use in men's soaps and hair care products, as in the bay rum that has enjoyed a certain popularity since Victorian times. The scent of bay is considered masculine, and bay is still an ingredient in many men's products today. Aromatherapists consider bay oil a good antiseptic for the respiratory system. Bay combines well with other essential oils, such as eucalyptus.

PARTS USED: Leaves

FOR HEALTH:

• The warm and stimulating scent of bay diffused into your environment may help relieve the discomfort of respiratory ailments and can be especially restorative when you are convalescing from a long illness.

• Apply a hot compress of a drop of bay diluted with a tablespoon of vegetable carrier oil to relieve arthritic pain.

• Bay is a natural insect repellent.

FOR BEAUTY:

• A few drops of bay oil in your shampoo may help control oily hair and dandruff.

• Bay oil is often used as a tonic to stimulate hair growth.

• Bay oil is used in men's colognes and soaps.

PRECAUTIONS:

Bay oil can be irritating to the skin and should never be applied in its pure state; in fact its chemical constituent, eugenol, is capable of corroding metal. Always dilute bay with a less irritating base carrier oil. When used correctly, bay is a safe and effective essential oil.

BENZOIN

(*Styrax benzoin*)

The essential oil of benzoin, which comes from the resin of benzoe trees in Asia, has anti-inflammatory and anti-septic qualities that make it useful in the treatment of asthma, bronchitis, coughs, and sore throats. Benzoin, with its warm vanilla scent, is also a good remedy for eczema and psoriasis, and is often a component of beauty treatments. The essential oil is a good fixative, since it does not evaporate as quickly as other essential oils. Benzoin combines well with geranium and rose.

PARTS USED: Resin

FOR HEALTH:

- For nighttime relief of respiratory complaints such as asthma, bronchitis, coughs, and sore throats, place a bowl of hot water containing one drop of eucalyptus and three drops of benzoin at your bedside.

- For respiratory relief, apply a hot compress of a drop of eucalyptus and four drops of benzoin diluted with a tablespoon of vegetable carrier oil to your chest.

FOR BEAUTY:

- Because of its fixative qualities, the essential oil of benzoin is widely used in perfumes.

- For dry or aging skin, dilute two or three drops of benzoin with a tablespoon of vegetable carrier oil and apply twice a day. This is moisturizing to the skin and may help brown age spots fade. Add several drops of freshly squeezed lemon to your formula if bleaching age spots is your objective. (Be sure to perform a skin test before use.)

- A few drops of benzoin in your shampoo may help control oily hair and dandruff.

PRECAUTIONS:

The essential oil of benzoin has been known to cause allergic reactions, so it is especially important to perform a skin test before use. Benzoin is otherwise a safe and effective essential oil.

BERGAMOT

(*Citrus auran var bergamia*)

Bergamot, a member of the citrus family, is a small pear-shaped fruit that is a hybrid of orange and lemon. Its essential oil has natural antiseptic qualities similar to those of lavender, and it is used by aromatherapists throughout Europe to treat skin, respiratory, and urinary tract infections.

All the citrus oils are also wonderful antidepressants, especially in the wintertime. The refreshing and uplifting scent of bergamot is used to relieve anxiety, stress, and depression, and it is the essential oil of bergamot that gives Earl Grey tea its unique flowery aroma. Bergamot combines well with angelica, cedar, chamomile, geranium, lavender, lemon, neroli, rose, and ylang-ylang.

PARTS USED: Rind of the fruit

FOR HEALTH:

- Bergamot is very balancing and may be diffused into the air, mixed with a massage oil, or added to your bath to promote calm and stability.

- Apply one drop of bergamot oil diluted with a teaspoon of vegetable carrier oil to a cold sore at the first sign of outbreak. An itching or tingling sensation usually precedes the actual cold sore.

- Several drops of bergamot oil diluted with a tablespoon of vegetable carrier oil may be topically applied to relieve eczema and psoriasis.

- For respiratory infections a few drops of bergamot may be diffused into your environment or mixed with vegetable carrier oil and rubbed on the chest.

- For urinary tract infections, add a drop or two of bergamot to a sitzbath. Use once a day.

FOR BEAUTY:

- Add several drops of the essential oils of bergamot and chamomile to a mild lotion and use to moisturize dry or chapped skin.

- Dilute one or two drops of bergamot and ylang-ylang with a teaspoon of vegetable carrier oil and give yourself a refreshing facial massage.

- For bad breath, add a drop of bergamot oil to a cup of water and use as a mouthwash.

PRECAUTIONS:

When applied topically, bergamot may increase your susceptibility to sunburn. If you use bergamot oil, limit your exposure to the sun. If this is impossible, choose an alternate essential oil.

Correct storage of bergamot oil is also important, as citrus oils are the quickest to evaporate. Keep the bottle tightly closed and store in a closet away from sunlight. The oil should be clear, as any cloudiness may indicate spoilage that can lead to skin problems.

When these simple precautions are followed, bergamot is a safe and effective essential oil.

BIRCH

(Betula allegheniesis)

The sharp and pungent essential oil of birch is useful for treating muscle pain, arthritis, and skin rashes. For these purposes it may be added to baths, massage oils, or compresses. Birch is often combined with wintergreen.

PARTS USED: Bark

FOR HEALTH:

- Dilute several drops of the essential oil of birch with a
  tablespoon of vegetable carrier oil and massage into
  aching muscles or joints.

- For skin rashes such as eczema and psoriasis, dilute
  three drops of birch with a tablespoon of vegetable
  carrier oil and apply to the affected areas twice a day.

- You may also add a few drops of birch to your bath or
  make a birch compress for these purposes.

FOR BEAUTY:

- Birch oil may be added to a shampoo to stimulate hair
  growth.

PRECAUTIONS:

Birch is generally a safe and effective essential oil.

CADE

(*Juniperus oxycedrus*)

The essential oil of cade, which comes from the juniper
tree, has been used by French aromatherapists since the
nineteenth century to treat skin problems. Today it is

most commonly used to strengthen hair and combat hair problems.

PARTS USED: Wood

FOR HEALTH:

- For skin rashes dilute several drops of cade with a tablespoon of vegetable carrier oil and apply once a day.

FOR BEAUTY:

- Add a few drops of cade to your shampoo to help control dandruff.

- Add cade to your shampoo or conditioner to strengthen damaged hair.

- Cade oil may be added to a shampoo to stimulate hair growth.

PRECAUTIONS:

Cade is generally a safe and effective essential oil.

CAJEPUT
(*Melaleuca leucadendron*)

The cajeput tree of the East Indies yields a pungent oil with a warm, camphorlike scent. Cajeput contains the chemical cineole, which is a natural stimulant to the central nervous system and also has strong antiseptic qualities. The healing properties of cajeput are particularly helpful in the treatment of respiratory problems, muscle aches and pains, digestive disorders, urinary tract infections, and skin diseases. Cajeput combines well with eucalyptus, mint, and wintergreen.

PARTS USED: Leaves and branches

FOR HEALTH:

- Cajeput may be diffused into the air to ease congested breathing due to colds, coughs, bronchitis, flu, and sinus infections.

- A combination of several drops of cajeput diluted with a tablespoon of vegetable carrier oil may also reduce inflammation and ease breathing difficulties. Massage the chest with this preparation several times a day.

- A massage oil containing cajeput may ease muscle aches and pains.

- For digestive problems such as stomachache and diarrhea, place a hot cajeput compress on your stomach, or massage the stomach area with several drops of the essential oils of cajeput diluted with a tablespoon of vegetable carrier oil.

- For urinary tract infections, use gentle circular motions to rub a cajeput-based massage oil into the abdomen and kidney region in the lower back.

- For skin problems such as acne, eczema, or psoriasis, dilute several drops of cajeput with a tablespoon of vegetable carrier oil and apply to the affected areas twice a day.

- Cajeput is a natural insect repellent.

FOR BEAUTY:

- To reduce the appearance of skin eruptions that may increase as you age, apply two or three drops of cajeput diluted with a tablespoon of vegetable carrier oil. Use twice a day as needed.

PRECAUTIONS:

Cajeput is generally a safe and effective essential oil.

CALENDULA

(*Calendula officinalis*)

Calendula, which is distilled from marigold petals, has a long and distinguished history in the tradition of natural healing. Garlands of calendula or marigolds were once festooned around doorways to promote good health and prevent illness from entering the home. In aromatherapy today calendula is most often used to heal wounds and burns.

PARTS USED: Flowers

FOR HEALTH:

- Apply a hot calendula compress to a wound to stop bleeding and promote healing.

- A drop or two of calendula oil blended in a mild lotion may soothe mild burns and calm inflamed skin conditions.

- To speed the healing of bruises, apply a cool compress made with several drops of calendula diluted with a tablespoon of vegetable carrier oil. Use up to three times daily.

- To relieve a painful earache, dip a cotton swab in calendula oil and place in the ear overnight.

- Apply a drop of undiluted calendula to a cold sore or other herpes lesion at the first sign of an outbreak.

- Dilute several drops of the essential oil of calendula with a tablespoon of vegetable carrier oil and gently massage over your varicose veins. Do not apply pressure to the affected veins.

FOR BEAUTY:

- Add a drop of calendula oil to a mild lotion to formulate an effective treatment for sensitive or acne-prone skin.

- A calendula compress may also be a helpful remedy for broken capillaries or spider veins.

PRECAUTIONS:

Because of its stimulating qualities, experts recommend that calendula be strictly avoided during pregnancy. Otherwise calendula is generally a safe and effective essential oil.

CAMPHOR

(*Cinnamomum camphora*)

Camphor is a strong and stimulating essential oil that was once the primary ingredient in smelling salts. Although we are now well past the Victorian era and no

longer require camphor to relieve swoons, vapors, and
fainting spells, this essential oil is still valued for its
strengthening effect on the nervous system. Its aroma is
similar in pungency to that of eucalyptus, and camphor
is related to cinnamon as well. Because camphor is such
a powerful scent, only small amounts should be used.

PARTS USED: Wood

FOR HEALTH:

• Diffuse a drop of camphor oil into your environment
for a strengthening effect on the nervous system.

• Because it regulates overactive sebaceous glands,
camphor oil can be a useful treatment for acne. Once
a day apply a cotton swab lightly dipped in undiluted
camphor oil directly on pimples. The most convenient
application is just before bedtime.

• Camphor has antiseptic qualities, and diffusing a drop
into the air you breathe may help you ward off a cold.

PRECAUTIONS:

Because of its very strong and stimulating qualities, experts advise care in the use of camphor oil. If you are or
suspect you may be pregnant, or if you suffer from allergies or asthma, this is not the right essential oil for you.
Otherwise camphor is generally a safe and effective essential oil.

CARDAMOM

(*Elettaria cardamomum*)

The soft, warm, and spicy fragrance of cardamom played an important role in ancient Egyptian, Greek, and Roman perfumes. The Chinese considered cardamom an excellent remedy for all digestive disorders, and cardamom remains an essential ingredient today in many Asian cuisines. In aromatherapy cardamom is valued by women who experience fluid retention due to PMS or menopause. Its uplifting scent may also be an aid to concentration.

PARTS USED: Seeds

FOR HEALTH:

- Diffuse several drops of cardamom into the air to lift your spirits and stimulate memory and concentration.

- To relieve the water buildup and irritability that sometimes accompany PMS and menopause, use circular motions to massage the diluted essential oil of cardamom into the stomach and lower back.

PRECAUTIONS:

Cardamom is a hot oil and can easily sensitize the skin. Always use with a base oil. Cardamom is otherwise a generally safe and effective essential oil.

CARROT SEED

(*Daucus carota*)

Fresh carrots, so rich in beta-carotene, are among the healthiest vegetables you can eat. Eating carrots is good for your skin, and the essential oil of carrot seed is excellent for skin complaints. It is particularly helpful in moisturizing and revitalizing our skin as we grow older.

PARTS USED: Seeds

FOR BEAUTY:

- Massage dry skin, spider veins, and wrinkles with several drops of the rejuvenating essential oil of carrot seed diluted with a tablespoon of vegetable carrier oil. Use once a day at bedtime.

- Apply a cool compress to affected areas once a day.

PRECAUTIONS:

Carrot seed is generally a safe and effective essential oil.

CEDAR

(*Cedrus atlantica*)

Cedars are the trees most frequently mentioned in the Bible, and in ancient times they acted as a symbol of fertility. In fact the warm and woody scent of cedar is still used today in men's preparations to promote sexual stimulation. Modern aromatherapists also use cedar to tone the respiratory system. Cedar combines well with bergamot, jasmine, juniper, neroli, and rose.

PARTS USED: Wood

FOR HEALTH:

- Cedar and rosemary may be diffused into the environment to enhance sexuality.

- Inhaling the steam of cedar oil may have a beneficial effect on the respiratory system.

- Cedar is a natural insect repellent.

FOR BEAUTY:

- Cedar is a stimulant, and products that contain cedar may act as helpful toners for oily skin.

- A few drops of cedar oil in your shampoo may help control oily hair and dandruff.

- Cedar is often used as a tonic to stimulate hair growth.

PRECAUTIONS:

Because of its stimulating qualities, experts recommend that cedar be strictly avoided during pregnancy. Otherwise cedar is generally a safe and effective essential oil.

CELERY

(*Apium graveolens*)

Celery has diuretic qualities that were first noted by Hippocrates, the Father of Medicine. Today celery juice is often drunk to counteract the fluid retention that accompanies PMS and menopause, while the essential oil may be added to your bath to relieve nervous fatigue. Legend also has it that celery possesses aphrodisiac qualities.

PARTS USED: Seeds

FOR HEALTH:

- The pungent aroma of several drops of celery oil in your bath can act as a pick-me-up after a long day at the office.

- The stimulating quality of celery oil in your bath or diffused through an aroma lamp may act as a sexual stimulant.

- To relieve uncomfortably chilled hands or feet, increase circulation by adding a few drops of celery oil to a bowl of hot water and treat yourself to a long soak.

PRECAUTIONS:

Celery is generally a safe and effective essential oil.

CHAMOMILE

(Chamaemelum nobile or *Matricaria chamomila)*

Chamomile is one of the safest and most effective essential oils. Alongside lavender, it has traditionally been cultivated for its medicinal uses and is used in European hospitals to purify and disinfect the air.

Chamomile contains a high proportion of naturally calming ester compounds and is an excellent remedy for nervous tension. It also possesses natural antispasmodic and anti-inflammatory properties, making chamomile a fine choice for the treatment of abdominal pain—ranging from a baby's colic to PMS—and stress-related headaches. Chamomile has traditionally played a major role in beauty as well as health, as women place cold wet chamomile teabags under their eyes to reduce puffiness, or rinse their hair with a combination of chamomile and lemon to brighten fair hair.

There are two main types of chamomile: *Chamaemelum nobile,* or Roman chamomile, and *Matricaria chamomila,* which is German chamomile. Both types are helpful in relieving nervous tension, but the more intense German variety is also particularly effective in treating problems such as inflammatory conditions, stomach ailments, and cold sores. German chamomile, with its intense blue color and strong hops smell, is easy to distinguish from Roman chamomile. The primary chemical constituent of German chamomile is the anti-inflammatory agent azulene.

One form of chamomile is sometimes preferable to the other, and when that happens, it is clearly marked as Roman or German in the list below. In other instances the functions of Roman and German chamomile overlap, and either type will do the trick. Chamomile is very compatible with other essential oils, including bergamot, geranium, lavender, lemon, melissa, and rose.

PARTS USED: Flowers

FOR HEALTH:

- The essential oil of chamomile may be diffused into the atmosphere, added to bathwater, or massaged into the body to dissolve nervous tension. It is an excellent remedy for everyday tension and stress.

- Roman chamomile is helpful in treating stress-related sinus headaches and migraines. Use your fingertips to lightly massage the diluted oil into the temples and sinus areas.

- Roman chamomile is used to treat the stomachaches, indigestion, and diarrhea that so often accompany stress. Dilute a few drops of Roman chamomile with a tablespoon of vegetable carrier oil and massage into the abdomen, using broad circular strokes. You can also make a hot Roman-chamomile compress and rest with it on your tummy, or add a few drops of the essential oil to your bath.

- Massage diluted Roman chamomile into affected areas to lessen muscle spasm.

- To relieve the water buildup and irritability of PMS, use circular motions to massage the diluted essential oil of Roman chamomile into the stomach and lower back.

- For baby's colic apply a warm Roman chamomile compress to the tummy.

- German chamomile is an excellent treatment for skin conditions such as acne and eczema. Dilute one to two drops of German chamomile with a tablespoon of the carrier oil calendula and apply to the affected areas.

- Apply a drop of undiluted German chamomile to a cold sore or other herpes lesion at the first sign of an outbreak.

- A cool German-chamomile compress may be applied to relieve the itching and stinging of insect bites or bee stings.

- To relieve baby's teething pain, dilute a drop of the essential oil of German chamomile with a tablespoon of vegetable carrier oil and rub a small amount directly on the gums.

- For earaches, dilute a drop of German chamomile with a teaspoon of vegetable carrier oil, dip a cotton swab in this mixture, and place the mixture in the ear overnight.

FOR BEAUTY:

- To reduce facial puffiness (especially underneath the eyes), apply a chamomile poultice. Steeped teabags will do the trick.

- To open and cleanse pores, make your own facial steambath. Add several drops of chamomile oil to a quart of hot water, cover your head with a towel, and rest your face about twelve inches above the bowl or pot. Make sure that the water is not too hot.

- Add a few drops of chamomile oil to your regular shampoo to lighten fair hair.

PRECAUTIONS:

Chamomile is a gentle and effective essential oil, so safe that it is considered the classic children's remedy.

Cinnamon

(*Cinnamomum ceylanicum* or *Cinnamomum cassia*)

Cinnamon, which originated in Sri Lanka, is one of the oldest spices in the world. Cinnamon oil, like the spice, is warm and stimulating. Aromatherapists today recommend cinnamon to stimulate circulation and speed recovery from colds.

PARTS USED: Leaves

FOR HEALTH:

- Use an aroma lamp to diffuse the warm and stimulating scent of cinnamon into the air. Cinnamon is particularly restorative when you have a deep chill or are recovering from an illness.

- A cool cinnamon compress may be applied to relieve the itching and stinging of insect bites or beestings.

- Cinnamon is a natural insect repellent.

FOR BEAUTY:

- Cinnamon was one of the ingredients of Carmelite water in the Middle Ages, and today it is often used in men's colognes and soaps.

PRECAUTIONS:

Cinnamon oil should be used with caution, as approximately 5 percent of people are allergic to it. Cinnamon oil can be irritating to the skin and should never be applied in its pure state; always dilute with vegetable carrier oil. Otherwise cinnamon is generally a safe and effective essential oil.

CITRONELLA

(*Cymbopogon nardus*)

Citronella, a member of the same tropical grass family as lemongrass and palmarosa, has a strong lemony scent that has traditionally been used as a natural insecticide. Citronella also has natural antiseptic qualities and may be applied to mosquito or other insect bites to relieve itching and swelling.

PARTS USED: Leaves

FOR HEALTH:

- Apply several drops of citronella oil diluted with a tablespoon of vegetable carrier oil to soothe the itching of insect bites.

- A few drops of citronella can act as an effective natural insect deterrent. Add to the melted wax surrounding a lit candlewick.

PRECAUTIONS:

Citronella is generally a safe and helpful essential oil. However, because it is inexpensive and has a pleasant aroma, citronella is sometimes used to adulterate more costly oils, such as geranium, rose, and verbena.

CLARY SAGE

(*Salvia sclarea*)

The essential oil of clary sage was valued by the ancient Egyptians as a shield against the plague, and later was prized by the Greeks for its ability to relax the nerves and improve the memory. Today the euphoric aroma of clary sage is used to relieve a wealth of conditions, especially those related to depression, stress, and fatigue.

Clary sage is one of the classic remedies for conditions specific to women: PMS, menstrual cramps, childbirth, and menopause. Since clary sage can help you get hold of runaway emotions, it is even a useful remedy for the postpartum baby blues. In fact clary sage is recommended to ease transitions of all kinds.

Clary sage is both physically and psychologically relaxing, and so it is very popular in holistic treatments. The sensual scent of clary sage also enjoys a certain reputation as an aphrodisiac. This very versatile essential oil combines well with bergamot, cypress, geranium, jasmine, lavender, and sandalwood.

PARTS USED: Flowers

FOR HEALTH:

• The essential oil of clary sage may be circulated through the air via an aroma lamp, ring, or diffuser to reduce stress, banish moodiness, and give a general lift to your spirits. Some feel that the aroma enhances creativity.

• Clary sage is the classic remedy for menstrual discomfort. Dilute several drops of the essential oil with a tablespoon of vegetable carrier oil and, using gentle circular motions, massage into your abdomen and lower back.

• This same massage oil can be used to relieve the water buildup and irritability that often accompany PMS and menopause.

• Add several drops of clary sage diluted in carrier oil to your bath to relieve premenstrual discomfort.

• Clary sage is a natural aphrodisiac for many people. Diffuse the essential oil through the air, add a few drops to your bath, or exchange slow and sensual massages with your partner, using several drops of clary sage diluted with a tablespoon of vegetable carrier oil.

• Some women find that massage with an oil containing several drops of clary sage and a drop of rose is helpful during labor.

- A bath with this essential oil can help relieve a case of postpartum baby blues.

- Clary sage, chamomile, and lavender may be combined on a cool compress and applied to the forehead, neck, and back of the head to ease migraine pain and discomfort.

- A clary sage bath can calm down a cranky child and help him (and you) get a good night's sleep.

FOR BEAUTY:

- The essential oil of clary sage has fixative qualities and is widely used in perfumes.

- A dilution of several drops of clary sage with a tablespoon of vegetable carrier oil can be used to condition damaged hair.

- For bad breath, add a drop of the essential oil of clary sage to a cup of water and use as a mouthwash.

PRECAUTIONS:

Experts recommend that clary sage not be used by those who suffer from epilepsy. Alcohol intake before or after clary sage can intensify its effects. Clary sage is otherwise a very safe and effective essential oil.

CLOVE
(*Caryophyllus aromaticus*)

Clove is a stimulating essential oil that has long been prized in China and India for its powerful healing qualities. More recently scientists have discovered that clove contains a high proportion of the chemical eugenol, which accounts for its antiseptic and analgesic qualities, and clove has become a common ingredient in many commercial toothpastes and mouthwashes. French aromatherapists have noted that the anti-inflammatory effects of clove make it a helpful treatment for arthritis.

PARTS USED: Flowers and leaves

FOR HEALTH:

- Apply a hot compress of a drop of clove diluted with a tablespoon of vegetable carrier oil to relieve arthritic pain.

- Diffuse the warm and stimulating scent of clove into the environment. Clove is particularly restorative when you are recovering from a long illness.

- The aroma of clove may act as an aphrodisiac.

- Use a drop of diluted clove oil on a cotton swab to numb the pain of a toothache. A brief application (less than a minute) should be sufficient. Longer use may lead to local irritation.

- To relieve uncomfortably chilled hands or feet, soak them for five minutes in a bowl of hot water infused with a drop or two of clove oil. Clove is a warming and stimulating oil.

- Clove is a natural insect repellent.

FOR BEAUTY:

- Whole cloves have traditionally been placed in oranges to make pomanders, a sweet and natural way to perfume your home around the holidays.

- Clove oil is often used in perfumes and soaps.

PRECAUTIONS:

Clove oil should be used with caution, as approximately 5 percent of people are allergic to it. Clove oil can be irritating to the skin and should never be applied in its pure state; in fact its chemical constituent eugenol is capable of corroding metal. Always dilute clove with vegetable carrier oil. When used correctly, clove is a safe and effective essential oil.

CYPRESS

(*Cupressus sempervirens*)

Cypress are tall evergreen trees that yield an essential oil with a smoky, woody fragrance. The Egyptians recorded the first medical uses of cypress on papyrus, and used cypress trees to make their sarcophagi. Later the Greek physician Hippocrates noted the natural astringent quality of cypress and recommended cypress oil for the treatment of hemorrhoids, and the oil is still used for this purpose today. Modern aromatherapists note the calming properties of cypress, especially in the reduction of menopausal tension. Cypress combines well with lavender, lemon, myrtle, and pine.

PARTS USED:　Leaves and cones

FOR HEALTH:

- The scent of cypress may be diffused into the air, mixed with a massage oil, or added to your bath to counteract the nervous tension associated with menopause.

- Dilute several drops of the essential oils of cypress and myrtle with a tablespoon of vegetable carrier oil and gently apply to hemorrhoids once daily.

- Gently massage varicose veins with an oil containing cypress. Do not apply pressure to the affected veins.

- To speed the healing of bruises, apply a cool compress made with several drops of cypress diluted with a tablespoon of vegetable carrier oil. Use up to three times daily.

- Add a few drops of the essential oil of cypress to your bath or shower to improve circulation. You can also pour a few drops onto a sponge or washcloth and lightly massage over hemorrhoids or varicose veins, lather and rinse.

- Inhaling the steam of cypress oil may have a beneficial effect on the respiratory system.

FOR BEAUTY:

- Since cypress oil may improve circulation, massage an oil containing cypress into skin disfigured by broken veins or capillaries.

- A cypress massage may be a helpful treatment for cellulite.

- Since cypress is a natural astringent, products that contain cypress may act as helpful toners for oily skin.

- A few drops of cypress oil in your shampoo may help control oily hair and dandruff.

PRECAUTIONS:

Cypress is generally a safe and effective essential oil.

EUCALYPTUS

(*Eucalyptus globulus, Eucalyptus radiata,* and *Eucalyptus citriodora*)

The eucalyptus tree yields a fresh and pungent oil with strong antibiotic and antiviral qualities. The healing qualities of eucalyptus, a natural expectorant, are particularly helpful in the treatment of respiratory problems such as colds, flu, and sinusitis. Eucalyptus also contains the chemicals eucalyptol and cineole, which stimulate the central nervous system.

There are hundreds of varieties of eucalyptus trees, which originated in Australia but are now found in countries around the world. *Eucalyptus globulus,* with its camphorlike aroma, yields the most effective healing essential oil, followed by *Eucalyptus radiata. Eucalyptus citriodora* emits a fresh, lemony scent that is used in perfumes and potpourri. In the list below, any type of eucalyptus can be used, although the greatest therapeutic value will be derived from *Eucalyptus globulus,* followed by *Eucalyptus radiata.* Eucalyptus is compatible with many other essential oils, including angelica, hyssop, lemon, pine, and thyme.

PARTS USED: Leaves and branches

FOR HEALTH:

- Eucalyptus may be inhaled several times a day to break up congestion due to colds, coughs, bronchitis, flu, and sinus infections. Add three drops to a quart of hot water, cover your head with a towel, and rest your face about twelve inches above the bowl or pot. Breathe deeply.

* A combination of several drops of eucalyptus diluted with a tablespoon of vegetable carrier oil and massaged into the chest several times a day may also reduce inflammation and ease breathing difficulties.

* Diffuse eucalyptus into the air or add a few drops to your bath to relieve congestion.

* Because of its extremely stimulating nature, a few drops of eucalyptus may be diffused through the air or added to a bath or massage oil to relieve mental and physical fatigue.

* A massage oil containing eucalyptus may ease the pain of arthritis.

* A drop or two of eucalyptus may be applied to cleanse minor cuts and scrapes.

* Because it regulates overactive sebaceous glands, eucalyptus oil is often a useful treatment for acne. Once a day apply a cotton swab lightly dipped in undiluted eucalyptus oil directly on pimples. The most convenient application is just before bedtime.

* A cold eucalyptus compress applied to the legs or feet can help bring down a fever.

- Combine eucalyptus with angelica in an aroma lamp, ring, or diffuser to prevent the spread of colds and viruses during flu season.

- Eucalyptus is a natural insect repellent.

FOR BEAUTY:

- Add a few drops of eucalyptus to your shampoo to help control dandruff.

PRECAUTIONS:

Eucalyptus is generally a safe and effective essential oil.

EVERLASTING

(*Helichrysum angustifolium* or *Helichrysum italicum*)

Everlasting, which is also known as everlast or immortelle, yields a reddish essential oil that is warm and spicy. Everlasting is grounding like other essential oils such as vetiver, but in a lighter and less intense way. It is similar to cypress in its calming characteristics.

Everlasting also has extremely effective anti-inflammatory properties, making it especially helpful in the treatment of hemorrhaging, bruising, and swelling. In addition it possesses antibacterial and antiviral qualities. Everlasting is compatible with many other essential oils, including bergamot, grapefruit, lemon, orange, neroli, verbena, and cypress.

PARTS USED: Flowers

FOR HEALTH:

- To speed the healing of bruises and swelling, apply a cool compress made with a drop or two of everlasting diluted with a tablespoon of vegetable carrier oil. Use up to three times daily.

- Dilute a drop or two of everlasting with a tablespoon of vegetable carrier oil and gently massage over your varicose veins. Do not apply pressure to the affected veins.

- A warm bath with diluted everlasting can be an invaluable aid for detoxification. Allow the consequences of a heavy meal or a late night out on the town to slowly seep out of your skin.

- A bath with everlasting may also be a very calming and grounding experience.

- Everlasting is a useful treatment for acne. Once a day apply a cotton swab lightly dipped in everlasting oil directly on pimples. The most convenient application is just before bedtime.

- Several drops of everlasting oil diluted with a tablespoon of vegetable carrier oil may be topically applied to relieve skin rashes such as eczema and psoriasis.

- For sunburn, mix several drops of everlasting in a tablespoon of St. John's wort oil and apply to affected areas.

- Everlasting may be inhaled several times a day to break up congestion due to colds, coughs, bronchitis, flu, and sinus infections. Add three drops to a quart of hot water, cover your head with a towel, and rest your face about twelve inches above the bowl or pot. Breathe deeply.

- A massage oil containing everlasting may relieve menstrual cramps.

PRECAUTIONS:

Everlasting is generally a safe and effective essential oil. Because it is an especially powerful oil, some aromatherapists recommend that you begin your journey into essential oils with less intense varieties and gradually work your way up to everlasting if necessary.

FENNEL
(*Foeniculum vulgare*)

Fennel, a favorite remedy of the ancient Egyptians and Chinese, is characterized by its strong licorice scent. The seeds have traditionally been used as a digestive aid, and aromatherapists use the essential oil made from fennel seeds to calm nervous tension and relieve muscle pain. Fennel combines well with rose and sandalwood.

PARTS USED: Seeds

FOR HEALTH:

• The essential oil of fennel is very calming and warming to the body and can be used to relieve stress and nervous tension. Fennel may be diffused into the air, mixed with a massage oil or mild lotion, or added to your bath to alleviate stress.

• Massage an oil containing fennel into sore muscles to relieve minor aches and pains.

• To improve digestion and strengthen the liver, apply a hot compress of several drops of fennel diluted with a tablespoon of vegetable carrier oil to the stomach.

• Fennel is very balancing for digestive problems such as constipation, diarrhea, and flatulence (gas). Use in a diffusion or massage oil.

• If you've overindulged last night and wake up with a hangover, add a few drops of fennel to your morning bath.

• Fennel is a natural insect repellent.

FOR BEAUTY:

• Fennel has qualities similar to natural hormones. To firm sagging skin and give it a more youthful appearance, dilute several drops of fennel with a tablespoon of carrier oil and use to massage your face and neck.

You may also add a few drops of fennel to a mild lotion and use it to moisturize your skin.

• A fennel massage may be a helpful treatment for cellulite.

• For bad breath, add a drop of fennel oil to a cup of water and use as a mouthwash.

PRECAUTIONS:

Fennel should generally be used with caution due to its high phenolic resin content. It should be avoided during pregnancy. Fennel is otherwise a safe and effective essential oil.

FRANKINCENSE

(Boswellia thurifera)

According to the Bible, frankincense was so valuable that, along with gold and myrrh, it was one of the gifts brought by the three kings to celebrate the birth of Jesus. The rich, warm scent of frankincense is still found in many churches today, and aromatherapists recommend the essential oil for its calming and grounding influence. Many find the woody aroma helpful for concentration during meditation and yoga. Frankincense may also ease breathing difficulties. It combines well with sandalwood.

PARTS USED: Resin

FOR HEALTH:

- The grounding aroma of frankincense may be diffused into the air, mixed with a massage oil or mild lotion, or added to your bath to promote calm.

- Frankincense may be inhaled several times a day to improve the lung and sinus congestion which accompanies respiratory infections. Add two drops to a quart of hot water, cover your head with a towel, and rest your face about twelve inches above the bowl or pot. Breathe deeply.

- Frankincense may also be used in this way to treat asthma, as it slows and deepens breathing.

- To reduce inflammation and relieve congestion, massage the sinus and chest areas with several drops of frankincense diluted with a tablespoon of vegetable carrier oil several times a day.

FOR BEAUTY:

- Frankincense has astringent qualities, and products that contain this essential oil may act as helpful toners for oily skin.

- To help smooth wrinkles and rejuvenate aging skin, massage each night with several drops of frankincense diluted with a tablespoon of vegetable carrier oil.

PRECAUTIONS:

Frankincense is generally a safe and effective essential oil.

GERANIUM

(*Pelargonium graveolens* and *Pelargonium odoratissimum*)

Geranium is one of the most versatile essential oils in aromatherapy. Its soft floral scent is very balancing, as it can both reduce stress and restore calm or dispel tiredness and stimulate energy. Geranium is said to lift your spirits, banish depression, and reduce nervous tension and fear.

The essential oil of geranium has physical as well as psychological benefits. A natural antiseptic, it is helpful in the treatment of a number of skin disorders. Geranium is an adrenal cortex stimulant, and because of this excels in its ability to balance the production of sebum. Geranium combines well with many other essential oils, including benzoin, bergamot, chamomile, clary sage, lemongrass, melissa, patchouli, and vetiver.

PARTS USED: Leaves

FOR HEALTH:

- Geranium has a flowery, balancing scent that may be diffused into the atmosphere to relieve stress, exhaustion, and depression. It is very useful when you are convalescing from a health problem such as the flu.

- For a refreshing pick-me-up, add a few drops of geranium to your bath.

- To relieve fatigue, dilute several drops of geranium with a tablespoon of vegetable carrier oil and massage into your neck and temples or stomach.

- For skin problems such as athlete's foot, eczema, hemorrhoids, insect bites and stings, or shingles, dilute five drops of geranium with a tablespoon of vegetable carrier oil. Apply twice a day.

- To speed the healing of bruises, apply a cool compress made with several drops of geranium diluted with a tablespoon of vegetable carrier oil. Use up to three times daily.

- To dispel the nausea and discomfort of a hangover, apply a cool geranium compress to your forehead and neck.

- Geranium is a natural insect repellent.

FOR BEAUTY:

- Many perfumes contain geranium.

- A geranium massage may be a beneficial treatment for cellulite, as it has diuretic properties and stimulates the lymph system. Its stimulating qualities also increase circulation.

PRECAUTIONS:

Geranium is generally a safe and helpful essential oil. However, since geranium is quite expensive to produce, it is often adulterated with less expensive (and also less effective) lemongrass. Be certain to buy geranium from a reputable store or practitioner, and be prepared to pay a relatively steep price in order to get the real thing.

GRAPEFRUIT
(*Citrus paradissi*)

Grapefruit, a member of the citrus family, is a fresh, light, and cheerful scent that is just right for lifting your spirits. All the citrus oils are wonderful antidepressants, especially in the wintertime. The stimulating aroma of grapefruit is said to relieve anxiety, stress, and depression. Grapefruit blends beautifully with lavender.

PARTS USED: Rind of the fruit

FOR HEALTH:

• The essential oil of grapefruit is very stimulating and can provide a welcome break when you are feeling overwhelmed by life. Grapefruit may be diffused into the air, mixed with a massage oil or mild lotion, or added to your bath to combat depression.

FOR BEAUTY:

- Grapefruit is a stimulant, and products that contain grapefruit may act as helpful toners for oily skin.

- Add a few drops of grapefruit to your shampoo to help control greasy hair.

- A grapefruit massage may be a beneficial treatment for cellulite, as its stimulating qualities increase circulation.

PRECAUTIONS:

When applied topically, grapefruit may increase your susceptibility to sunburn. Try to limit your exposure to the sun or use extra sun protection. Correct storage of grapefruit oil is also important, as citrus oils are the quickest to evaporate. Keep the bottle tightly closed and store in a closet away from sunlight. The oil should be clear, as any cloudiness may indicate spoilage that can lead to skin problems. When these simple precautions are followed, grapefruit is a safe and effective essential oil.

HYSSOP

(*Hysoppus officinalis*)

In ancient times hyssop was prized by the Romans both as a protection against the plague and for its aphrodisiac qualities. In this century French aromatherapists use anti-inflammatory hyssop as an inhalant to treat respiratory problems, since this essential oil acts as a natural decongestant, expectorant, and stimulant. Hyssop is compatible with a number of other essential oils, including clary sage, eucalyptus, lavender, pine, and rosemary.

PARTS USED: Flowers and leaves

FOR HEALTH:

- Hyssop may be diffused into the air to relieve the discomfort of colds, flu, and other respiratory ailments.

- Apply a hot hyssop compress to ease congestion and suppress coughs.

PRECAUTIONS:

Because of its stimulating qualities, hyssop should never be used by pregnant women or by those who have epilepsy. In France, where essential oils are used internally as well as externally, for safety's sake hyssop is available by prescription only. When used properly, however, hyssop is a safe and effective essential oil.

JASMINE

(*Jasminum officinale*)

The sweet floral aroma of jasmine is said to penetrate fear and depression and replace these negative emotions with optimism and at times even euphoria. Jasmine may be diffused through the air to resolve nervous tension and restore confidence, and is especially useful when connected with relationships. Its sensual aroma is reputed to inspire sensuality and act as an aphrodisiac; Cleopatra is said to have worn jasmine to seduce Mark Antony. Jasmine combines well with neroli, orange, patchouli, rose, and sandalwood.

PARTS USED: Flowers

FOR HEALTH:

* The relaxing and warming aroma of jasmine may be diffused into the atmosphere to relieve depression, low self-confidence, and sexual tension.

* While jasmine is most commonly diffused into the air, you may also add a few drops to your bath or dilute with a tablespoon of vegetable carrier oil and use in massages.

FOR BEAUTY:

* Many perfumes contain jasmine.

PRECAUTIONS:

Jasmine is generally a safe and effective essential oil. Yet it is also very costly because of the enormous amount of flowers necessary to produce a small amount of oil. Buyers should keep this in mind when purchasing a high-quality jasmine oil. Since it is a powerful oil, very little is needed for treatment. What looks like an inexpensive bargain in jasmine is more likely to be a synthetic or adulterated version with little therapeutic value. Be certain to buy the essential oil of jasmine from a reputable store or practitioner, so that you know you are getting the real thing.

JUNIPER

(*Juniperus communis*)

In the Middle Ages juniper was burned in the streets to prevent the spread of the plague. Its fresh, fruity scent is strengthening and uplifting and is used today to maintain focus during meditation. Aromatherapists value juniper for its natural antiseptic and diuretic qualities. It is invaluable for detoxification.

PARTS USED: Berries

FOR HEALTH:

• Juniper is very stimulating and may be inhaled to restore energy and strength.

- Juniper may be diffused into the air via an aroma lamp, ring, or diffuser to detoxify the environment and prevent the spread of germs in enclosed spaces.

- A juniper bath may be an invaluable aid for detoxification. Dilute several drops of the essential oil with a tablespoon of vegetable carrier oil and add to warm bathwater. Slowly soak away the aftermath of a heavy meal or a late night out on the town.

- Juniper can be a helpful treatment for acne or eczema. Dilute five drops of juniper with a tablespoon of vegetable carrier oil and apply several times a day.

- Massage diluted juniper into stiff joints and muscles to relieve everyday aches and pains.

- Add a few drops of juniper to your bath to help counteract the water buildup of PMS.

- Massage juniper-based oil into the legs to increase circulation and help reduce swelling or prevent the development of varicose veins.

- Add a few drops of juniper oil to a sitzbath if you suffer from vaginitis or a urinary tract infection. Use once a day. (Do *not* use for kidney infections.)

- Juniper is a natural insect repellent.

FOR BEAUTY:

- Add a few drops of juniper to a bowl of warm water to create a refreshing facial sauna for oily skin.

- A juniper massage may be a beneficial treatment for cellulite, as its stimulating qualities increase circulation.

PRECAUTIONS:

Because it may stimulate menstruation, juniper should never be used by pregnant women. It is also an inappropriate remedy for kidney problems. Juniper is otherwise a safe and effective essential oil.

LAUREL

(*Laurus nobilus*)

The laurel tree was a symbol of glory to the ancient Greeks, who believed that laurel would protect them not only from infectious disease but also from thunder and lightning. Aromatherapists today consider the essential oil of laurel to be a helpful treatment for respiratory problems and muscle aches and pains. Laurel contains the chemical eugenol, which has natural antiseptic and analgesic qualities.

PARTS USED: Leaves

FOR HEALTH:

- Diffuse the warm aroma of laurel into the air to relieve the discomfort of respiratory problems such as bronchitis or flu. Laurel is a natural expectorant.

- Add a few drops of laurel oil to your bath or apply a hot compress of a drop of laurel diluted with a tablespoon of vegetable carrier oil to relieve arthritic pain.

- A hot laurel compress can also be applied to conditions such as sprains, sore muscles, and stiff necks.

- A hot laurel compress on the abdomen may provide some comfort during an episode of diarrhea.

FOR BEAUTY:

- The essential oil of laurel is often used in soaps, lotions, and perfumes.

- Laurel may be used as a tonic to stimulate hair growth.

PRECAUTIONS:

Laurel contains the chemical eugenol, which in its pure state is capable of corroding metal. Laurel can be irritating to the skin and should always be diluted with vegetable carrier oil. When used correctly, however, laurel is a safe and effective essential oil.

LAVANDIN

(*Lavandula fragrans*)

The essential oil of lavandin is a hybrid of two species of
wild lavender. Lavandin is often mistakenly sold as lavender, for it is much easier to produce and far less expensive than the essential oil of true lavender. It can
easily be distinguished from true lavender by its distinctive sweet fragrance. Lavandin has a mildly calming effect which is reminiscent of lavender, and may be used
as a bath oil or home fragrance.

PARTS USED: Leaves

FOR HEALTH:

• A lavandin bath or a diffusion of lavandin in your
  home may have a pleasant, calming effect.

FOR BEAUTY:

• Lavandin is a common ingredient in inexpensive
  soaps and perfumes.

PRECAUTIONS:

Lavandin is a safe, pleasant, and mildly effective essential oil. The difficulty is that lavandin is not nearly as
useful as lavender, yet it is often sold under that name.
(Also see Lavender.)

LAVENDER

(*Lavandula angustifolia, Lavandula officinalis,* and *Lavandula vera*)

Lavender is one of the world's most popular essential oils. It is also one of the most versatile oils in aromatherapy, with properties ranging from analgesic to antiseptic to antidepressant to antispasmodic to antibacterial to sedative, making it the virtual Swiss Army knife of essential oils.

The founder of twentieth-century aromatherapy, French scientist Dr. René-Maurice Gattefossé, accidentally discovered the healing properties of lavender when he severely burned his hand in a laboratory experiment and instantly plunged it into a nearby bowl of liquid, which happened to be pure lavender oil. The pain was relieved and the burn quickly healed.

Lavender has long been used in European hospital rooms to purify and disinfect the air. The region of Provence in France is famous for its lavender fields, as is Surrey, England, where a company called Yardley discovered lavender in the 1800s and began adding it to their soaps and perfumes.

In this country, women often add a few drops of lavender to their baths to relieve stress and anxiety, or diffuse lavender into the air to get a good night's sleep. Lavender has a high ester content that gives it a natural calming effect on the nervous system and renders it especially useful in relieving muscle spasm. In addition high concentrations of linalol make the oil very antiseptic. It is a very balancing essential oil that may relieve nervousness, restore equilibrium, and promote stability.

There are several varieties of lavender. Most lavender available today is *Lavandula angustifolia,* which comes from large wild lavender plants. *Lavandula officinalis,* which is a smaller and more powerful medicinal plant used by aromatherapists, is difficult to produce, very expensive, and rarely available; it grows in the high Alpine regions of the Mediterranean and thus is harder to cultivate. *Lavandula vera,* or true lavender, is basically equivalent to *Lavandula officinalis.* All types of lavender have varying degrees of the same qualities and are very compatible with other essential oils including chamomile, clary sage, neroli, rose, and ylang-ylang.

PARTS USED: Leaves

FOR HEALTH:

- Lavender is very cooling. Applied topically, a few drops of undiluted lavender may speed the healing of burns. It takes the heat out of a burn almost immediately and accelerates cellular regeneration so that wounds heal more readily.

- Treat insect bites, bee stings, and other minor injuries with a drop of undiluted lavender oil.

- A combination of lavender and aloe vera can take the sting out of a painful sunburn.

- To speed the healing of bruises, apply a cool compress made with several drops of lavender diluted with a tablespoon of vegetable carrier oil. Use up to three times daily.

- Several drops of lavender oil diluted with a table-spoon of vegetable carrier oil may be topically applied to relieve skin rashes.

- Because it regulates sebaceous glands, lavender is a helpful treatment for acne. Very pure lavender has a high concentration of linalol, which makes it very anti-septic. Once a day apply a cotton swab lightly dipped in undiluted lavender oil directly on pimples. The most convenient application is just before bedtime.

- The essential oil of lavender may be diffused with ner-oli or rose to relieve insomnia and help you get a good night's sleep. You can also place a few drops of laven-der on your pillow to help induce sleep.

- Lavender is very calming and may be inhaled to bal-ance mood swings and promote stability.

- Water infused with lavender can be gently massaged into the temples to soothe headache pain, especially if you are suffering from a migraine. Slowly circle your temples with your fingertips. Chamomile and clary sage may also be combined with lavender on a cool compress and applied to the forehead, neck, and back of the head to ease migraine pain and discomfort.

- Massage diluted lavender into affected areas to re-lieve muscle spasm.

- Add a few drops of lavender oil to a sitzbath if you suffer from vaginitis or a urinary tract infection. Use once a day.

- Massage lavender-based oil into the legs to increase circulation and help reduce the swelling or prevent the development of varicose veins.

- Diffuse naturally antiseptic lavender into the environment to help prevent the spread of germs in sickrooms and other enclosed spaces.

- Spritzing with hydrolats during a flight or road trip is a terrific way to keep skin moisturized and feel refreshed overall. The antiseptic and calming qualities of lavender water are especially useful during long flights, when stale air is constantly recirculated. You can also moisten a tissue or handkerchief with a drop or two of lavender oil and simply keep it close at hand.

- After a long trip add a few drops of lavender and ylang-ylang oils to your bath to relieve jet lag and help you get a good night's sleep.

- A lavender bath can provide comfort and relief after any stressful experience and is especially useful if you suffer from chronic anxiety or high blood pressure.

- Lavender is a natural insect repellent.

FOR BEAUTY:

- The delicate perfume of lavender has been used since ancient times, when Romans added it to their baths.

- Regular use of lavender hydrolats (floral waters) on the face can eliminate or reduce redness and blotchiness. Hydrolats may also calm overactive and oily skin conditions.

- To help rejuvenate aging skin, massage each night with several drops of lavender diluted with a tablespoon of vegetable carrier oil.

- Massage diluted lavender oil into your abdomen, using gentle circular motions, to prevent stretch marks during and after pregnancy or extreme weight loss.

- Lavender water has astringent qualities that can help tone and tighten the skin. To make a floral water for greasy skin, add two drops of lavender and three drops of bergamot to an ounce of pure spring water.

- Add several drops of lavender to a mild shampoo to help control oily hair.

- A few drops of lavender oil in a warm bath may be a beneficial treatment for cellulite. Rub the skin first with a loofah (a rough sponge) to stimulate circulation.

- For bad breath, add a drop of lavender to a cup of water and use as a mouthwash.

PRECAUTIONS:

Lavender is a gentle and effective essential oil. It is one of the few essential oils that is so safe it may even be used undiluted for many healing purposes. Unfortunately because lavender is so popular that it is most people's first essential oil, and lavender is also very expensive to produce, it is often adulterated with other oils. Be certain to buy lavender from a reputable store or practitioner so that you know you are getting the real thing. (Also see Lavandin.)

LEMON

(*Citrus limon*)

The essential oil of lemon possesses a light, refreshing scent, and lemons and oranges are the two citrus oils most commonly used in aromatherapy. The stimulating scent of lemon oil is said to aid concentration, lift your spirits, and relieve fatigue. Like all the citrus oils, lemon is a wonderful antidepressant, especially in the wintertime. Lemon also has powerful antibacterial properties, which make it useful in treating cuts and wounds. Lemon combines well with other essential oils such as cedar, eucalyptus, fennel, juniper, lavender, and pine.

PARTS USED: Skin of the fruit

FOR HEALTH:

• Light, citrusy lemon has antibacterial qualities and may be circulated through the air via an aroma lamp, ring, or diffuser to prevent the spread of germs or to detoxify the environment of smoke and other heavy odors. It is particularly useful in neutralizing unpleasant odors in a patient's room.

- Lemon is balancing to the nervous system and may be diffused into the atmosphere to relieve depression and mental fatigue and to increase concentration.

- Apply a drop of slightly diluted lemon oil to relieve the itch and swelling of insect bites.

- Combine a drop of lemon with a teaspoon of the carrier oil arnica to clean cuts and wounds and stop them from bleeding.

- For eczema and other itchy skin conditions, take a sponge bath using several drops of lemon oil diluted with a quart of water.

- Add a drop of lemon to massage oils to increase their effectiveness in easing muscle aches and pains.

- Massage diluted lemon oil into your abdomen, using gentle circular motions, to relieve menstrual pain.

- To relieve hot flashes, apply a cold lemon compress. Dip a cotton towel or washcloth into a bowl of cold water with four to six drops of the essential oil.

FOR BEAUTY:

- For bad breath, add a drop of lemon to a cup of water and use as a mouthwash.

- Massage diluted lemon oil into your abdomen, using gentle circular motions, to help prevent stretch marks during pregnancy.

- To help age spots fade, dilute two or three drops of lemon with a tablespoon of vegetable carrier oil and apply twice a day.

- Lemon oil has astringent qualities that can help tone and tighten the skin. This may be particularly useful in treating large-pored, oily skin.

- A lemon massage may be a beneficial treatment for cellulite.

- Add a few drops of lemon to your shampoo to brighten fair hair.

PRECAUTIONS:

Lemon oil may cause skin irritation. Always use diluted, and never more concentrated than a 1 percent solution.

When applying lemon oil to your skin, use extra care in your sun protection. Exposure to sunlight or ultraviolet light after use may cause a skin rash.

Correct storage of lemon oil is also important; keep the bottle tightly closed and store in a closet away from sunlight. The oil should be clear, as any cloudiness may indicate spoilage that can lead to skin problems.

When these simple precautions are followed, lemon is a safe and effective essential oil.

LEMONGRASS

(*Cymbopogon citratus*)

Lemongrass, a member of the same fragrant tropical-grass family as citronella and palmarosa, has a strong, uplifting lemony scent that has long been prized in the Ayurvedic medicine of India. Lemongrass is balancing and calming to the nervous system and may increase your powers of concentration. In addition it is said to stimulate digestion and milk production in nursing mothers. Lemongrass combines well with eucalyptus, geranium, juniper, lavender, lime, and pine.

PARTS USED: Grass

FOR HEALTH:

- Use a revitalizing mixture of lemongrass and rosemary in your bath each morning, especially if you are overtired and need an extra lift to face the day ahead.

- Diffuse lemongrass into the air around you to relieve fatigue and increase concentration.

- For jet lag after a long trip, take a bath with lemongrass diluted with carrier oil to help relieve mental and physical fatigue.

- Lemongrass may be circulated through the air via an aroma lamp, ring, or diffuser to prevent the spread of germs and detoxify it of smoke and other heavy odors.

- Several drops of lemongrass oil diluted with warm water can act as a natural and pleasant-smelling insect deterrent.

FOR BEAUTY:

- The antiseptic properties of lemongrass, along with its clean, fresh scent, make it a common ingredient in soaps.

- Lemongrass has astringent qualities, and products that contain lemongrass may help tone and tighten oily skin.

PRECAUTIONS:

The essential oil of lemongrass may irritate sensitive skin, so it is especially important to perform a skin test before use. Also, since lemongrass is relatively inexpensive and has a pleasant aroma, it is sometimes used to adulterate more costly oils such as geranium, rose, and verbena. Lemongrass is otherwise a safe and effective essential oil.

LIME
(*Citrus limetta*)

Limes have a long history of usefulness in health. In the age of exploration they were given to English sailors to prevent scurvy, which resulted in the not altogether correct (or intentionally flattering) English nickname "Limeys."

Lime, a member of the citrus family, has a sweet and tangy aroma that is refreshing and energizing. Its stimulating scent can help you improve your memory and concentration as you prepare a report for work or balance your monthly bank statement. Lime also has antiseptic qualities that can disinfect and purify the air around you. All the citrus oils are wonderful antidepressants, especially in the wintertime. Lime combines well with bergamot, cedar, clary sage, lemongrass, and pine.

PARTS USED: Skin of the fruit

FOR HEALTH:

- The essential oil of lime is lively and refreshing. Diffuse lime into your environment to relieve exhaustion and fatigue and give a special lift to your spirits.

- Circulate the fresh scent of lime through the air via an aroma lamp, ring, or diffuser to prevent the spread of germs and detoxify the environment of smoke and other heavy odors.

FOR BEAUTY:

- Lime is a stimulant, and products that contain lime may act as helpful toners for oily skin.

- A few drops of lime oil in a warm bath may be a helpful treatment for cellulite. Rub the skin first with a loofah to stimulate circulation.

- A lime massage may also be a beneficial treatment for cellulite.

PRECAUTIONS:

As with lemon, extra caution must be exercised in sun protection after you apply lime oil to your skin. Exposure to sunlight or ultraviolet light after use may cause a skin rash. Correct storage of lime oil is also important; keep the bottle tightly closed and store in a closet away from sunlight. Lime is otherwise a safe and effective essential oil.

MARJORAM

(*Origanum marjorana*)

The essential oil of marjoram has a long and versatile history in natural healing. Its sweet and spicy aroma is used to ease stress and anxiety and may be diffused into the air to help you get a good night's sleep. Marjoram has a naturally calming and relaxing effect on the nervous system, which makes it especially useful in treating a number of health concerns related to nervous tension, such as anorexia, diarrhea, flatulence, insomnia, high blood pressure, PMS, menopause, migraines, and muscle aches and pains.

Marjoram has often been confused with oregano, which is a member of the marjoram family. Yet oregano is far more pungent than marjoram, and the relaxing and calming properties of marjoram are greater than those of oregano. Marjoram combines well with bergamot and lavender.

PARTS USED: Branches

FOR HEALTH:

- The scent of marjoram is very warming and calming. Diffuse the aroma into the air, mix with a massage oil, or add to your bath to relieve depression, anxiety, and insomnia, and to promote calm and stability.

- Marjoram can also be used in these ways to counteract the nervous tension associated with PMS and menopause.

- A marjoram bath can provide comfort and relief after any stressful experience and is especially useful if you suffer from chronic anxiety or high blood pressure.

- To stimulate appetite and reduce the stress connected with anorexia, diffuse several drops of marjoram into your environment, add a few drops to your bath, or use a marjoram-based massage oil to rub stomach, hands, and feet.

- Mix a few drops of marjoram in a tablespoon of vegetable carrier oil and gently rub into the temples to soothe a migraine.

- Apply a hot compress made with several drops of marjoram diluted with a tablespoon of vegetable carrier oil to stimulate circulation and relieve sore or aching muscles.

- A hot marjoram compress on the abdomen may provide comfort during episodes of diarrhea or flatulence.

- To relieve a painful earache, dilute a drop of marjoram with a teaspoon of vegetable carrier oil, dip a cotton swab in this mixture, and place the mixture in the ear overnight.

- To speed the healing of bruises, apply a cool compress made with several drops of marjoram diluted with a tablespoon of vegetable carrier oil. Use up to three times daily.

- To relieve gum infections and sore throats, add a drop of marjoram to a cup of water and use as a mouthwash.

- The aroma of marjoram may discourage sexual desire.

PRECAUTIONS:

Because of its stimulating qualities, marjoram should never be used by pregnant women. Marjoram is otherwise a generally safe and effective essential oil.

MELISSA
(*Melissa officinalis*)

Melissa, which is also known as balm or lemon balm, was a primary ingredient in the famous Carmelite water used by nuns in seventeenth-century France. Today the essential oil of melissa, with its fresh, light citrus fragrance, is used to soothe nervous tension, irritability, or depression. If you suffer from insomnia, try adding a few drops of oil to water in which you wash your bed linen, or tuck several crushed leaves into your pillowcase. Melissa also has strong antiviral properties, and may help clear up the blisters of herpes simplex. It combines well with geranium, lavender, myrtle, neroli, and rose.

PARTS USED: Leaves

FOR HEALTH:

• Diffuse the essential oil of melissa into your environment to counteract the effects of daily stress and anxiety.

• To stimulate appetite and reduce the stress connected with anorexia, diffuse several drops of melissa into the environment, add a few drops to your bath, or use a melissa-based massage oil to rub stomach, hands, and feet.

• Apply one drop of melissa oil diluted with a teaspoon of vegetable carrier oil to a cold sore at the first sign of outbreak. An itching or tingling sensation usually precedes the actual cold sore.

• Mix two drops each of melissa and rose in a tablespoon of vegetable carrier oil and gently rub into the temples to soothe a migraine.

• Use an aroma lamp or add a few drops of melissa to your bath to relieve the symptoms of asthma.

FOR BEAUTY:

- Melissa may be used in perfumes, as it was in Carmelite water in the Middle Ages.

PRECAUTIONS:

Melissa oil may cause skin irritation. Always use diluted, and never more concentrated than a 1 percent solution. It's also important to purchase the *pure* essential oil. Melissa or balm oil is often made from the much less expensive (and also less effective) citronella. Be certain to buy melissa from a reputable store or practitioner, and be prepared to pay a relatively steep price in order to get the real thing. Melissa is otherwise a very safe and effective essential oil.

MYRRH

(*Commiphora myrrha*)

Myrrh was an ingredient in incense used by ancient Egyptians, and along with frankincense and gold was reputed to be one of the special gifts of the Magi to the baby Jesus. Today the warm, smoky scent of myrrh is still considered helpful for meditation, and aromatherapists recommend the naturally antiseptic essential oil for skin and mouth problems.

PARTS USED: Resin

FOR HEALTH:

- The essential oil of myrrh may be diffused into the air to lift your spirits and help you focus during meditation.

- For inflamed skin problems such as acne, eczema, and scars, massage the affected areas with several drops of myrrh diluted with a tablespoon of vegetable carrier oil.

- Mouthwashes containing myrrh are available in many health food stores. Gargle with a mouthwash containing myrrh if you experience toothaches, bleeding gums, canker sores, or bad breath. You may also create your own mouthwash by adding a drop of myrrh to a cup of water. (Do not swallow.)

FOR BEAUTY:

- Myrrh has astringent qualities, and products that contain this essential oil may act as helpful toners for oily skin.

- To help rejuvenate aging skin, massage each night with several drops of myrrh diluted with a tablespoon of vegetable carrier oil.

PRECAUTIONS:

Myrrh is generally a safe and effective essential oil.

MYRTLE

(*Myrtus communis*)

Myrtle has long been a symbol of purity, and today its fresh, camphorlike scent continues to be valued for its ability to cleanse the mind and body. Myrtle has natural antiseptic qualities that make it particularly useful in caring for the skin, as well as astringent properties that make it helpful in the treatment of hemorrhoids. Myrtle combines well with cypress, lavender, lemon, neroli, and pine.

PARTS USED: Leaves

FOR HEALTH:

- Circulate the fresh scent of myrtle through the air via an aroma lamp, ring, or diffuser to cleanse the mind and spirit and strengthen focus during meditation.

- Dilute several drops of myrtle with a tablespoon of vegetable carrier oil and use a moist gauze pad to apply to the blemishes of acne.

- Dilute several drops of the essential oils of myrtle and cypress with a tablespoon of vegetable carrier oil and gently apply to hemorrhoids once daily.

- To treat conjunctivitis, spritz a myrtle hydrolat onto a cotton pad and place over the eyelid. Alternatively dampen the cotton pad, add a drop of myrtle, and place on the eyelid. (Never apply this or any other essential oil directly into the eyes.)

• To relieve the pain and speed the healing of insect bites and stings and shingles, apply a mixture of eight drops of myrtle diluted with a tablespoon of vegetable carrier oil.

• Myrtle is a natural insect repellent.

FOR BEAUTY:

• Since myrtle is a natural astringent, products that contain myrtle may act as helpful toners for oily skin.

PRECAUTIONS:

Myrtle is generally a safe and effective essential oil.

NEROLI

(*Citrus aurantium bugardia*)

The sweet floral aroma of neroli is often diffused through the air to relieve nervous tension and fatigue and to lift your spirits. The most important use of neroli is in psychoaromatherapy, in treating problems in the emotional sphere such as anxiety and depression.

The essential oil of neroli is extracted from the flowers of orange trees, and it takes virtually a ton of flowers to produce a mere quart of oil. Neroli is named after the

Princess of Nerole, who introduced orange-blossom oil to Italy in the 1600s. All the citrus oils are wonderful antidepressants, especially in the wintertime. Neroli also enjoys a certain reputation as an aphrodisiac.

PARTS USED: Flowers

FOR HEALTH:

- Neroli is tranquilizing and balancing to the nervous system and may be diffused into the atmosphere to relieve depression, tension, and anxiety.

- Massage several drops of neroli diluted with a table-spoon of vegetable carrier oil into your abdomen, us-ing gentle circular motions, to relieve stress.

- Add a few drops of neroli to an evening bath to help get a good night's sleep.

- To decompress after a tough day at the office, lie down and relax with a hot neroli compress on your tummy.

- Neroli can also be used in all of the above ways— diffused into the air or added to a bath, massage oil, or hot compress—to relieve premenstrual tension.

FOR BEAUTY:

- Neroli has qualities similar to natural hormones. To firm sagging skin, speed up the growth of new skin cells, and give skin a more youthful appearance, dilute several drops of neroli with a tablespoon of carrier oil and use to massage your face and neck. You may also add a few drops of neroli to a mild lotion and use it to moisturize your skin.

• A neroli massage may be a helpful treatment for preventing stretch marks during pregnancy.

• To treat acne, make your own facial steambath by adding three drops of neroli to a quart of hot water. Cover your head with a towel and rest your face about twelve inches above the pot. Make sure that the water is not too hot.

• A neroli compress may act as a helpful remedy for broken capillaries or spider veins.

PRECAUTIONS:

When applied topically, neroli may increase your susceptibility to sunburn. Try to limit your exposure to the sun or use extra sun protection. Correct storage of neroli oil is also important, as citrus oils are the quickest to evaporate. Keep the bottle tightly closed and store in a closet away from sunlight. The oil should be clear, as any cloudiness may indicate spoilage that can lead to skin problems. When these simple precautions are followed, neroli is a safe and effective essential oil.

NIAOULI

(*Melaleuca viridiflora*)

Niaouli, a member of the myrtle family, yields an anti-septic oil that is valued for its use in the treatment of respiratory and urinary tract infections. Niaouli is compatible with many other essential oils, including eucalyptus, hyssop, lemon, myrtle, orange, and pine.

PARTS USED: Leaves

FOR HEALTH:

• Niaouli may be combined with eucalyptus and inhaled several times a day to improve lung and sinus congestion due to colds, coughs, bronchitis, flu, and sinus infections. Add two drops of niaouli and one drop of eucalyptus to a quart of hot water, cover your head with a towel, and rest your face about twelve inches above the bowl or pot. Breathe deeply.

• A combination of several drops of niaouli diluted with a tablespoon of vegetable carrier oil may also ease breathing difficulties. Massage the chest with this preparation several times a day.

• Use gentle circular motions to rub a niaouli-based massage oil into the abdomen when you suffer from a urinary tract infection.

- Diffuse niaouli into the air to relieve congestion.

- Add a few drops of niaouli and eucalyptus to an aroma lamp, ring, or diffuser to prevent the spread of colds and viruses during flu season.

PRECAUTIONS:

Niaouli is generally a safe and effective essential oil.

ORANGE

(*Citrus aurantium*)

The essential oil of orange possesses a sweet, warm scent that reduces stress and is both calming and uplifting. In ancient Rome, oranges were valued for their digestive qualities, and more recently French aromatherapists have recommended orange oil for gas, indigestion, and constipation. All the citrus oils are wonderful antidepressants, especially in the wintertime. The cheerful scent of orange is considered particularly appropriate for children.

PARTS USED: Skin of the fruit

FOR HEALTH:

- A sweet orange aroma may be circulated through the air via an aroma lamp, ring, or diffuser to reduce stress, improve your mood, or help you calm down and get a good night's sleep.

- For eczema and other itchy skin conditions, take a sponge bath using several drops of orange oil diluted with a quart of water.

- Add a drop of orange to massage oils to increase their effectiveness in easing muscle aches and pains.

- Orange is a safe and cheerful scent to add a little sunshine and purify the air of a child's room.

FOR BEAUTY:

- A few drops of orange oil in a warm bath may be a beneficial treatment for cellulite. Rub the skin first with a loofah to stimulate circulation. An orange-oil-based massage may also help.

- A massage oil containing orange may increase circulation and enliven aging skin.

PRECAUTIONS:

Extra sun protection is a must after applying orange oil, as your skin is more vulnerable to sun damage after use. Correct storage of orange oil is important, as citrus oils are the quickest to evaporate. Keep in tightly closed dark bottles away from sunlight. The oil should be clear, as any cloudiness may indicate spoilage that can lead to skin problems. When these simple precautions are followed, orange is a safe and effective essential oil.

PALMAROSA

(*Cymbopogon martini*)

Palmarosa, a member of the same fragrant tropical-grass family as citronella and lemongrass, has a sweet scent that is uplifting and regenerating. Palmarosa is a helpful treatment for a wide range of skin conditions, ranging from acne to aging skin. In addition the antiseptic qualities of palmarosa make this essential oil helpful in relieving the muscle discomfort that so often accompanies fevers and flu.

PARTS USED: Grass

FOR HEALTH:

- To treat acne, dilute several drops of the essential oil of palmarosa with a tablespoon of vegetable carrier oil and use a moist gauze pad to massage into blemishes once a day at bedtime.

- To relieve the aching muscles of flus and fevers, dilute five drops of palmarosa with a tablespoon of vegetable carrier oil and massage into the chest, shoulders, and neck.

- Add a few drops of palmarosa to your bath to revitalize your mood.

- Diffuse palmarosa into the air around you to refresh your spirits.

FOR BEAUTY:

- To add moisture and reduce the appearance of the wrinkles and spider veins of aging skin, dilute several drops of the essential oil of palmarosa with a tablespoon of vegetable carrier oil and use a moist gauze pad to massage into skin once daily at bedtime.

PRECAUTIONS:

Palmarosa is generally a safe and effective essential oil.

PATCHOULI

(*Pogostemon cablin*)

This woody, musky essential oil has played an important role in traditional Chinese medicine, and in aromatherapy today its natural antiseptic qualities make it especially helpful in the treatment of many skin conditions. The earthy scent of patchouli is also said to act as an aphrodisiac and combines well with bergamot, clary sage, geranium, jasmine, palmarosa, and ylang-ylang.

PARTS USED: Leaves

FOR HEALTH:

- To treat skin conditions such as acne, eczema, impetigo, and seborrhea, dilute several drops of patchouli with a tablespoon of vegetable carrier oil and use a moist gauze pad to gently apply to affected skin.

- To capture the aphrodisiac qualities of patchouli, diffuse into the air or add a few drops to your bath, massage oil, or mild body lotion.

- Patchouli is a natural insect repellent.

FOR BEAUTY:

- Because of its musky scent and fixative qualities, the essential oil of patchouli is widely used in perfumes.

- To rejuvenate aging skin, add a few drops of patchouli to a mild lotion or vegetable carrier oil and gently massage into the skin.

- To control dandruff, add a few drops of patchouli to a tablespoon of vegetable carrier oil and massage into your scalp several hours or the night before shampooing. Cover with a towel.

- To help condition dry, dark hair and keep it shiny, add a drop of patchouli and a drop of ylang-ylang to a tablespoon of vegetable carrier oil and apply to hair. Wrap hair in a warm towel and leave for an hour before shampooing.

PRECAUTIONS:

Patchouli is generally a safe and effective essential oil.

PEPPERMINT

(*Mentha piperita*)

Peppermint oil contains a substance that is known to relax the stomach and has traditionally been used to counteract digestive problems such as nausea and diarrhea. A whiff of peppermint oil may stave off an attack of motion or travel sickness. Other uses for peppermint include colds and flu.

PARTS USED: Leaves

FOR HEALTH:

- Carry a small bottle of peppermint oil when you travel if you or your child are prone to motion sickness. A sniff of peppermint (from the bottle, or on a tissue or handkerchief for your child) may prevent or cure nausea and discomfort.

- The essential oil of peppermint may be circulated through the air via an aroma lamp, ring, or diffuser to lessen gas, stomachache, nausea, vomiting, heartburn, and diarrhea.

- A small inhalation of peppermint oil is also safe enough to relieve morning sickness during pregnancy. Place several drops on a handkerchief or tissue and keep it in your pocket or purse to inhale as needed.

- To relieve digestive problems, massage the stomach region with a few drops of peppermint diluted with a tablespoon of vegetable carrier oil.

- To ease migraine pain, massage stimulating diluted peppermint into the temples and back of the neck.

- Add a few drops of peppermint oil to a bowl of hot water and breathe deeply to clear your sinuses when you are congested due to a cold or flu.

- Peppermint is good to use for its cooling effect on feverish conditions.

- Add a drop of peppermint and a drop of rose to your morning bath to relieve the nausea, headache, and general discomfort of a hangover. Always use in diluted form since peppermint is a sensitizing oil.

- To relieve the itching and discomfort of shingles, add a few drops of peppermint to a mild lotion and apply to the affected areas.

- Add a drop of peppermint oil to a cup of water and use as a mouthwash.

- To relieve the pain of a toothache, place a drop of peppermint oil on a sterile cotton swab and press gently against the affected area.

- Peppermint is a natural insect repellent.

FOR BEAUTY:

• To open and cleanse your pores, make your own facial steambath. Add five drops of peppermint oil to a quart of hot water, cover your head with a towel, and rest your face about twelve inches above the bowl or pot. Make sure that the water is not too hot.

PRECAUTIONS:

Peppermint is a sensitizing oil and should always be diluted before use. Peppermint is otherwise a safe and effective essential oil.

PETITGRAIN

(*Citrus aurantium bigaradia*)

The fresh, floral aroma of petitgrain is revitalizing and stimulating. The qualities of petitgrain are similar to the much more expensive neroli. Its relaxing and balancing fragrance is often diffused through the air or added to massage oils and baths to relieve nervous tension and fatigue and to prevent insomnia. The effect of petitgrain is to give you a lift when you are feeling down in the dumps. Like neroli, the most important use of petitgrain is in psychoaromatherapy, where it is used to treat emotional problems such as tension and sadness.

PARTS USED: Leaves, twigs, and unripe fruit

FOR HEALTH:

• Petitgrain is tranquilizing and balancing to the nervous system and may be diffused into your environment to relieve tension and calm anxiety.

• Add a few drops of petitgrain to your evening bath to prevent insomnia and help you get a good night's sleep.

• To relieve nervous tension and fatigue, massage several drops of petitgrain diluted with a tablespoon of vegetable carrier oil into your abdomen, lower back, chest, neck, hands, and feet.

FOR BEAUTY:

• To treat skin problems such as acne, make your own facial steambath by adding a drop of petitgrain to a quart of hot water. Cover your head with a towel and rest your face about twelve inches above the pot. Make sure the water is not too hot.

PRECAUTIONS:

When applied topically, petitgrain may increase your susceptibility to sunburn. Try to limit your exposure to the sun or use extra sun protection. Correct storage of petitgrain is also important, as citrus oils are the quickest to evaporate. Store in tightly closed dark bottles away from sunlight. The oil should be clear, as any cloudiness may indicate spoilage that can lead to skin problems. When these simple precautions are followed, petitgrain is a safe and effective essential oil.

PINE

(*Pinus sylvestris*)

The white-pine tree yields a stimulating, fresh, and pungent oil with strong antiseptic qualities. The healing abilities of this essential oil are particularly helpful in the treatment of respiratory problems, while its antibacterial properties make it useful for cleaning and disinfecting the air. Pine is compatible with a number of other essential oils, including angelica, cypress, eucalyptus, lemon, and myrtle.

PARTS USED: Needles, cones, and branches

FOR HEALTH:

• Pine may be inhaled at the first sign of a cold or flu.

• You may also dilute several drops of the essential oil with a tablespoon of vegetable carrier oil and massage into the chest. (Try substituting cypress, eucalyptus, or hyssop for two of the pine drops to create an even more effective synergistic remedy.)

• Apply a hot pine compress to the chest at the first sign of infection.

• Pine may be circulated through the air via an aroma lamp, ring, or diffuser to prevent the spread of germs or to detoxify it of smoke and other heavy odors.

- Create a massage oil containing several drops of pine diluted with a tablespoon of vegetable carrier oil. Rub into sore muscles to relieve minor aches and pains.

- A pine massage may ease the pain of arthritis.

- For urinary tract infections or vaginitis, add a few drops of essential pine oil to the bath. Alternatively, massage the diluted oil in circles around the stomach area.

- Pine is a natural insect repellent.

PRECAUTIONS:

For respiratory complaints, it is best to use pine as an inhalation. Pine is less often used as a massage oil, because it can irritate the skin. Be certain to perform a skin test before using pine. Pine is otherwise a generally safe and effective essential oil.

ROSE

(Rosa centifolia, Rosa damascena, and Rosa gallica)

From Cupid to Romeo and Juliet, rich and deeply fragrant roses are the stuff of legend. Rose is one of the world's favorite perfumes and is among the most popular, versatile, and precious essential oils. It takes two thousand pounds of petals to yield one pound of rose oil.

Rose is a wonderful balancing remedy for stress, depression, and insomnia, and many women find it especially helpful during PMS and menopause. It is a classic remedy for depression related to grieving. In addition rose is a good remedy for a wide range of health concerns, from migraines to sore throats.

There are hundreds of types of roses and rose hybrids. The damask rose, or *Rosa damascena,* originated in Syria and is now cultivated in Bulgaria and other countries around the world. The essential oil that is distilled from highly perfumed damask roses is known as otto or attar, and this is the rose oil with the greatest therapeutic value. Since it requires a great number of these roses to produce a very small amount of the essential oil, rose otto is also quite expensive.

In France the essential oil of *Rosa centifolia,* the cabbage rose, is a by-product of the manufacture of its famous rosewater, which itself is a wonderful skin tonic. The prolific *Rosa gallica* from Turkey has a heavy fragrance that many find to be overwhelming. Rose is very compatible with other essential oils, such as jasmine, lavender, neroli, and sandalwood.

PARTS USED: Petals

FOR HEALTH:

• Rose is mostly used in psychoaromatherapy today, to help us cope with our emotions.

• To relieve depression (especially when it is related to grieving), stress, or the tension that sometimes accompanies PMS and menopause, dilute several drops of the essential oil of rose with a tablespoon of vegetable carrier oil and, using gentle circular motions, massage into your abdomen, lower back, temples, and neck.

- The essential oil of rose—alone, or in combination with lavender or neroli—may be diffused into the air of your bedroom to help you get a good night's sleep.

- A rose bath can be very soothing and calming, especially to those who naturally have a somewhat nervous nature.

- Rose oil is a natural aphrodisiac for many people. Diffuse the essential oil through the air, add a few drops to your bath, or exchange slow and sensual massages with your partner, using several drops of rose diluted with a tablespoon of vegetable carrier oil.

- Mix two drops each of rose and melissa in a tablespoon of vegetable carrier oil and gently rub into the temples to soothe migraine pain.

- Add a drop each of rose and peppermint to your morning bath to relieve the nausea, headache, and general discomfort of a hangover.

- For eczema and psoriasis, apply a cool rose compress to affected areas.

- If you suffer from pruritus (anal itch), prepare a warm sitzbath with one drop each of rose and peppermint in a bowl of warm water. Use once a day.

- Some women find that massage with an oil containing several drops of clary sage and a drop of rose is helpful during labor.

- To relieve swollen, tired eyes, apply a cool rose compress.

- For sore throats, gargle with a drop of rose oil mixed in a cup of water.

- For bad breath or sores in the mouth, add a drop of rose oil to a cup of water and use as a mouthwash.

FOR BEAUTY:

- The rich and full-bodied aroma of rose is a classic ingredient in many perfumes.

- To help rejuvenate aging skin, massage each night with several drops of rose diluted with a tablespoon of vegetable carrier oil.

PRECAUTIONS:

Rose is a safe, versatile, and very effective essential oil. Unfortunately because rose is so expensive to produce, it is often adulterated with other oils. Be certain to buy the essential oil of rose from a reputable store or practitioner so that you know you are getting the real thing.

ROSEMARY

(*Rosemary officinalis*)

Long ago Hippocrates, the Father of Medicine, prescribed rosemary for the relief of liver disorders. Later in history rosemary, like angelica, was burned as incense during the plague in an attempt to capture its antiseptic qualities. Rosemary contains cineole, a substance that stimulates the central nervous system, and aromatherapists today diffuse the essential oil of rosemary into the environment to combat tiredness and depression.

PARTS USED: Flowers

FOR HEALTH:

- Because of its stimulating qualities, rosemary may relieve mental and physical fatigue. Use an aroma lamp, ring, or diffuser to disperse rosemary into the air, add a few drops to your bath, or mix rosemary into a massage oil.

- Treat yourself to a revitalizing rosemary bath each morning, especially if you are overtired and need an extra lift to face the day ahead.

- To stimulate digestion, massage your liver and stomach area with a combination of two drops each of the essential oils of rosemary and chamomile diluted with a tablespoon of vegetable carrier oil.

- For constipation, massage the lower abdomen in a circular clockwise direction with an oil containing rosemary.

- A drop or two of the essential oil of rosemary diluted with a tablespoon of vegetable carrier oil may be applied to the chest to ease breathing problems.

- Try massaging oil containing rosemary into sore muscles to relieve minor aches and pains. Use the base carrier oil arnica, which has natural anti-inflammatory properties of its own. Rub this mixture into sore muscles to increase local circulation and help remove lactic acid and cellular waste products.

- Diluted rosemary oil may be gently rubbed into the temples to relieve headaches, especially migraines.

- Add a few drops of rosemary to your bath to stimulate the elimination of toxins through your skin.

- A few drops of rosemary oil in the bath can be a helpful treatment for skin blemishes and rashes.

- Rosemary is a natural insect repellent.

FOR BEAUTY:

- Rosemary regenerates cells, increases local circulation, and is stimulating to the scalp. Dilute several drops in a nutritive carrier oil such as jojoba or camellia to help control dandruff.

- Rosemary is often used as a tonic to stimulate hair growth.

- Rosemary oil can help condition dark hair and keep it shiny.

- Rosemary is often used in perfumes.

- Rosemary is a stimulant, and products that contain rosemary may act as helpful toners for oily skin.

- A rosemary massage may be a beneficial treatment for cellulite, as the stimulating qualities of rosemary increase circulation. A few drops of rosemary in your bathwater may also be helpful.

PRECAUTIONS:

Because of its stimulating qualities, experts recommend that it be used with caution during pregnancy. Otherwise rosemary is generally a safe and effective essential oil.

SANDALWOOD

(*Santalum album*)

The heavy, sweet scent of sandalwood is grounding and balancing. Genuine sandalwood comes from the Mysore region of India and is a key feature of Ayurvedic medicine in that country. Sandalwood may be diffused through the air to reduce stress and to help you retain your focus in exercises such as meditation and yoga. Its exotic aroma is said to act as an aphrodisiac. Sandalwood combines well with benzoin, frankincense, jasmine, lemon, rose, and verbena.

PARTS USED: Wood

FOR HEALTH:

• Sandalwood has a very comforting, grounding woody scent that may be diffused into the atmosphere to relieve stress.

• Sandalwood is a natural aphrodisiac for many people. Diffuse the essential oil through the air, add a few drops to your bath, or exchange slow and sensual massages with your partner, using several drops of sandalwood diluted with a tablespoon of vegetable carrier oil.

• To relieve a sore throat, gargle with a drop of sandalwood oil mixed in a cup of water.

• For urinary tract infections, use gentle circular motions to rub a massage oil containing sandalwood into the abdomen and kidney region in the lower back.

FOR BEAUTY:

• Sandalwood is a classic ingredient in Asian perfumes.

PRECAUTIONS:

Sandalwood is generally a safe and effective essential oil.

TANGERINE

(*Citrus reticulata*)

The essential oil of tangerine has a lively, fresh scent that is cheerful and strengthening. Like oranges, tangerines have traditionally been noted for their digestive qualities. But in aromatherapy today, tangerine is more commonly used to relieve stress, anxiety, tension, and insomnia. All the citrus oils are wonderful antidepressants, especially in the wintertime. The cheerful scent of tangerine is considered especially appropriate for children.

PARTS USED: Skin of the fruit

FOR HEALTH:

- A sweet tangerine scent may be circulated through the air via an aroma lamp, ring, or diffuser to reduce stress, improve your mood, dispel sadness and irritability, and help you get a good night's sleep.

- Tangerine can be diffused into the air—or added to a bath, massage oil, or hot compress—to relieve premenstrual tension.

- Tangerine is a safe and cheerful scent to add a little sunshine and purify the air of a child's room.

PRECAUTIONS:

Extra sun protection is a must after applying tangerine oil, as your skin is more vulnerable to sun damage after use. Correct storage of tangerine oil is important; keep the bottle tightly closed and store in a closet away from sunlight. The oil should be clear, as any cloudiness may indicate spoilage that can lead to skin problems. When these simple precautions are followed, tangerine is a safe and effective essential oil.

TEA TREE

(*Melaleuca alterifolia*)

Tea tree oil is a popular first-aid remedy in Australia, where it has long been known for its antibacterial, antiviral, and antifungal properties. Studies in Australia, the United States, and England have verified the germ-fighting abilities of tea tree. In aromatherapy its essential oil is commonly used to treat small cuts and abrasions.

PARTS USED: Leaves

FOR HEALTH:

- Apply a drop of neat (undiluted) tea tree oil to cuts and scrapes to promote healing.

- Apply a drop of undiluted tea tree oil to a cold sore or other herpes lesions at the first sign of an outbreak.

- Tea tree oil can also be applied undiluted, in small amounts, to athlete's foot.

- A cool tea tree compress may be applied to relieve the pain of insect bites.

- Both French and American studies have shown that tea tree has potential in treating vaginal yeast infections.

PRECAUTIONS:

Tea tree is generally a safe and effective essential oil.

THYME

(*Thymus vulgaris*)

Thyme has strong antibacterial and antiviral characteristics, and has long been prized for its natural healing qualities. The essential oil is hot, stimulating and intense. In World War I, before the advent of modern antibiotics, an active constituent of thyme—thymol—was widely used to treat wounded soldiers. Aromatherapists today recommend thyme for a wide variety of conditions, including acne and other skin problems, respiratory ailments, anorexia, and muscle aches. Thyme oil is often used in combination with eucalyptus; it is very potent and must always be diluted before use.

PARTS USED: Leaves and flowers

FOR HEALTH:

- Diluted thyme oil may be inhaled several times a day to improve lung and sinus congestion due to colds, coughs, bronchitis, flu, and sinus infections. Thyme is a natural expectorant. Add one or two drops to a quart of hot water, cover your head with a towel, and rest your face about twelve inches above the bowl or pot. Breathe deeply.

- A combination of one or two drops of thyme diluted with a tablespoon of vegetable carrier oil may also ease breathing difficulties. Massage the chest with this preparation several times a day.

- Thyme is a natural astringent and is a component of many acne remedies.

- Add a drop or two of thyme oil to your bath to ward off depression and fatigue.

- A hot thyme and eucalyptus bath may soothe tired and aching muscles.

- To stimulate appetite and reduce the stress connected with anorexia, diffuse several drops of thyme into the environment, add a drop or two to your bath, or dilute one or two drops of thyme with a tablespoon of vegetable carrier oil and massage into stomach, hands, and feet.

- A drop or two of slightly diluted thyme oil may be applied to athlete's foot.

- A drop of thyme oil added to a mild lotion may be used to disinfect minor cuts and scrapes.

- A cool thyme compress may be applied to relieve the itching and stinging of insect bites or bee stings.

- A hot thyme compress on the abdomen may provide comfort during a bout of diarrhea.

- Disperse thyme oil through an aroma lamp, ring, or diffuser to prevent the spread of colds and viruses during flu season.

- Thyme is a natural insect repellent.

FOR BEAUTY:

- Add a drop of thyme to your shampoo to help control dandruff.

PRECAUTIONS:

The essential oil of thyme should be used with caution, as it can be extremely irritating to the skin. Thyme oil should never be applied in its pure state; always dilute with vegetable carrier oil. Because of its stimulating qualities, thyme should never be used by pregnant women or by those who have high blood pressure or epilepsy. Thyme is otherwise a safe and effective essential oil.

VANILLA
(*Vanilla planifolia*)

The sweet, warm, and distinctive scent of vanilla is calming and relaxing. Vanilla may be circulated through the air to reduce stress and irritability. It can foster communication by defusing tension and anger with its soft scent. Vanilla combines well with bergamot, lime, and rose.

PARTS USED: Pods

FOR HEALTH:

- Vanilla has a sweet fragrance that may be diffused into the atmosphere to relieve stress.

- You may also add a few drops of vanilla to your bath or to a mild body lotion. Breathe deeply and you will find that a sense of calm and serenity will gradually come to replace negative emotions such as irritability and frustration.

FOR BEAUTY:

- Vanilla is a very popular ingredient in perfumes, lotions, creams, bath gels, and other commercial products.

PRECAUTIONS:

Vanilla is generally a safe and effective essential oil.

VERBENA

(*Aloysia citriodora, Lippia citriodora,* or *Verbena triphylla*)

Verbena, which is also known as lemon verbena, has a strong lemony scent that is refreshing and stimulating. Ancient Egyptians used verbena in many women's remedies, while one of its Latin names comes from the seventeenth-century Italian scientist Augustin Lippi, who was the first European to identify the health benefits of verbena.

All the citrus oils are wonderful antidepressants, especially in the wintertime. The fresh citrus fragrance of verbena may be diffused into the air to relieve tiredness and depression and to increase concentration. Verbena also has strong antiseptic properties, which may make it useful in clearing up skin problems such as acne. This essential oil combines well with cedar, hyssop, jasmine, juniper, myrtle, neroli, and orange.

PARTS USED: Leaves

FOR HEALTH:

- Diffuse the essential oil of verbena into your environment to counteract the effects of tiredness and depression.

- After gently cleansing skin with a mild soap, dilute several drops of verbena with a tablespoon of vegetable carrier oil and use a moist gauze pad to apply to the blemishes of acne.

- Massage the diluted oil of verbena into muscles to loosen them before a workout, or to ease sore muscles afterward.

FOR BEAUTY:

- Verbena is often used in perfumes and soaps.

PRECAUTIONS:

The essential oil of verbena may irritate sensitive skin, so it is especially important to perform a skin test before use. Also since verbena is an expensive oil to produce, it is often adulterated with less expensive oils such as lemongrass and citronella. Verbena is otherwise a safe and effective essential oil.

VETIVER

(Vetiveria zizanoides)

The essential oil of vetiver, made from grass cultivated in Haiti and Indonesia, has a warm, earthy, peppery aroma that is prized in perfumes. The scent acts as a very deep and grounding force on nervous dispositions. In addition the physical effect of vetiver is thought to resemble that of estrogen, so it may be particularly helpful for women going through menopause or suffering from postpartum depression, when estrogen levels are apt to be low.

Since vetiver is such a powerful scent, only a very small amount is necessary to be effective. It is also quite possible that vetiver may not agree with you; the distinctive musty scent is loved by some and reviled by others. Vetiver combines well with cardamom, frankincense, jasmine, orange, neroli, rose, sandalwood, verbena, and ylang-ylang.

PARTS USED: Grass

FOR HEALTH:

- To reduce nervous tension and stress, add a drop of vetiver to your bath or disperse a drop of the scent into the air via an aroma lamp, ring, or diffuser.

- To help balance your mood during menopause and keep your changing life in balance, add a drop of vetiver to your bath, massage oil, or aroma lamp.

- A drop of vetiver in your bath may help you fend off a bout of postpartum depression.

- Vetiver is a natural insect repellent.

FOR BEAUTY:

- Vetiver is a popular ingredient in many perfumes.

- For aging skin, add a drop of vetiver to a mild lotion, or create a massage oil by diluting one drop with vegetable carrier oil.

PRECAUTIONS:

Vetiver is generally a safe and helpful essential oil. However, since vetiver is expensive to produce, it is often adulterated with less expensive (and also less effective) oils. Be certain to buy vetiver from a reputable store or practitioner and be prepared to pay a relatively steep price in order to get the real thing.

YARROW

(*Achillea millefolium*)

Yarrow was thought by the ancient Chinese to bring the two opposing forces of hard yang and soft yin into balance. Aromatherapists today continue to use yarrow as a balancing essential oil, especially during periods of transition in life, such as menopause.

The essential oil of yarrow contains active constituents such as azulene, camphor, eugenol, salicylic acid, and tannins, which are anti-inflammatory and speed the healing of wounds. Yarrow has a wide variety of uses, from regulating the menstrual cycle to easing headache pain. Its botanical name stems from the legend surrounding Achilles, who was said to use yarrow to mend the tendon in his heel. Yarrow combines well with other essential oils, including clary sage, cypress, melissa, and myrtle.

PARTS USED: Flowers, leaves, and stems

FOR HEALTH:

- During menopause women can use yarrow to help keep their changing lives in balance. Add a few drops of yarrow to your bath or disperse the scent into the air via an aroma lamp, ring, or diffuser.

- Because of its content of azulene, an anti-inflammatory agent, yarrow may be a helpful treatment for skin rashes. Apply a cool yarrow compress to affected areas.

- Massage a small amount of oil containing yarrow into the temples to relieve headache pain.

- A yarrow-based massage oil or lotion can be used to increase circulation and reduce the swelling of varicose veins.

- A yarrow sitzbath may be a helpful remedy for hemorrhoids or vaginal infections. Dilute three drops of yar-

row oil (and a drop of cypress, too, if you like) with
two cups of rosewater.

FOR BEAUTY:

• A mild lotion containing a drop of yarrow is a good
treatment for sensitive or acne-prone skin.

• Yarrow is often used as a tonic to stimulate hair
growth.

PRECAUTIONS:

When applying yarrow to your skin, use extra care in
your sun protection. Exposure to sunlight or ultraviolet
light after use may cause a skin rash. Yarrow also contains the chemical eugenol, which in its pure state is
capable of corroding metal; yarrow should always be diluted with vegetable carrier oil. When used correctly,
however, yarrow is a safe and effective essential oil.

YLANG-YLANG

(Cananga odorata)

Ylang-ylang, a tropical Asian tree that originated in the
Philippines, yields one of the quintessential women's
remedies in aromatherapy. Its intense, sweet, flowery
scent is balancing and restorative, gentle and soothing.
Ylang-ylang can relieve depression and may even correct
hormonal imbalances. Baths or massages with ylang-

ylang can reduce stress and anxiety and thus are useful adjunct treatments to regulate blood pressure and the mood swings of PMS. Ylang-ylang is often used in combination with complementary essential oils, such as bergamot, clary sage, lavender, and neroli.

PARTS USED: Flowers

FOR HEALTH:

- Add several drops of ylang-ylang to your bath to restore calm and promote relaxation.

- Combine ylang-ylang with a drop of lavender or clary sage in your bath to offset the mood swings of PMS.

- Ylang-ylang is very balancing and may be diffused into the air through an aroma lamp to reduce stress and anxiety.

- Dilute several drops of ylang-ylang in a tablespoon of a base vegetable oil and treat yourself to a massage. This massage may be especially helpful during labor.

- The scent of ylang-ylang can act as an aphrodisiac. If you are too tense to relax sexually, take a leisurely ylang-ylang bath or ask your partner to give you a gentle massage with the slightly diluted essential oil.

- A ylang-ylang bath may be useful in lifting all sorts of depression, including postpartum.

- After a long trip add a few drops each of ylang-ylang and lavender oils to your bath to relieve jet lag and help you get a good night's sleep.

FOR BEAUTY:

- For bad breath add a drop of ylang-ylang to a cup of water and use as a mouthwash.

- Ylang-ylang has a heady aroma and is often used in perfumes.

- Add a drop or two of ylang-ylang to your shampoo to condition hair and reduce split ends.

- To help condition dry dark hair and keep it shiny, add a drop of ylang-ylang and a drop of patchouli to a tablespoon of vegetable carrier oil and apply to hair. Wrap hair in a warm towel and leave for an hour before shampooing.

- Dilute one or two drops of ylang-ylang and bergamot with a teaspoon of vegetable carrier oil and give yourself a refreshing facial massage.

- Add a drop or two of ylang-ylang to a gentle skin lotion to help nourish and moisturize sensitive or aging skin. It helps regulate sebum production.

PRECAUTIONS:

Ylang-ylang is generally a safe and effective essential oil.

CHAPTER FOUR

AROMATHERAPY FOR HEALTH AND BEAUTY

The following is an A to Z guide to common health and beauty concerns and the essential oils that can help you manage them most effectively. Aromatherapy, like other holistic treatments, encourages your body to draw on its own natural healing and regenerative resources.

Synergy is an idea that will come up from time to time in this chapter. This simply means that at times mixing two or more essential oils creates a more powerful healing influence than a single oil could achieve on its own. In some cases a specific carrier oil—such as arnica, calendula, or St. John's wort—is also recommended. Many carrier oils have therapeutic benefits of their own that blend well with certain essential oils in the treatment of specific health and beauty problems. (See p. 17 in Chapter 2.)

Aromatherapy is a valuable complement to regular care, but it is by no means a replacement for it. When treating serious ailments, and in cases where your body does not respond to supportive aromatherapy, it is best to consult your medical practitioner.

Each profile will include:

* A description of the health or beauty concern

* How aromatherapy can help

ACNE

While it is most common during adolescence, acne can occur at any age and is probably linked to hormonal factors. Many women experience acne during PMS, and anyone can develop a few embarrassing blemishes when hormones are released as a result of chronic stress. If you have acne-prone skin, aromatherapy is best to use on a preventive basis. Some remedies can aggravate an active flare-up or broken skin.

Many essential oils can help you control acne. The most effective ones are juniper, lavender, and tea tree. Others include bergamot, cajeput, calendula, camphor, German chamomile, cypress, eucalyptus, everlasting, geranium, mint, myrrh, myrtle, neroli, palmarosa, patchouli, peppermint, petitgrain, rosemary, sage, thyme, and verbena. Try one essential oil at a time for approximately a month until you find the one that works best for you. (Be sure to perform a skin test first.)

AROMATHERAPY FOR ACNE:

- One of the best ways to maintain clear, healthy skin is to spray the face regularly with hydrolats (floral waters). Spritzing with a hydrolat is particularly helpful since you don't aggravate an active outbreak of acne by touching skin that is already sensitive or damaged. Lavender, which is naturally antiseptic and anti-inflammatory, is beneficial for all types of skin, especially overactive skin that produces large amounts of sebum. Spritz your entire face with a lavender hydrolat, or spritz a small quantity onto a cotton pad, add three to four drops of face oil (essential oil diluted with carrier oil), and gently pat your face with it.

- After gently cleansing skin with a mild soap, dilute several drops of an essential oil with a tablespoon of a light, astringent carrier oil that is noncomedogenic (one that won't clog your pores). Hazelnut and apricot are good carrier oils for this purpose, but your best option is probably squalene; squalene is an oil made from olives that has properties similar to human sebum. Use a moist cotton or gauze pad to apply to blemishes and gently blot to remove excess oil.

- Another good preventive measure is a facial steambath. You can make your own by adding three to five drops of an essential oil to a quart of hot water. Cover your head with a towel and rest your face about twelve inches above the pot. Make sure that the water is not too hot. (Do not use facial steambaths when skin is already badly broken out, since steam creates—and can spread—bacteria.)

- Certain essential oils may be applied with care during active acne outbreaks. Once a day apply a cotton swab lightly dipped in one drop of undiluted camphor, eucalyptus, or lavender oil directly on pimples. The most convenient application is just before bedtime.

AGING SKIN

Your skin undergoes many changes as you age. As estrogen production slows, sebaceous or sweat glands grow smaller and less effective. As a result sebum production slows and skin grows increasingly dry. Wrinkles, age spots, and spider veins may develop, facial tone grows duller, and skin is often less elastic.

Fortunately aromatherapy offers many strategies you can use to care for your skin as you age. Many essential oils act as natural moisturizers to revive lusterless skin, while others have rejuvenating properties that mimic those of natural hormones and can give skin a more youthful appearance. Essential oils such as lemon can help age spots fade.

AROMATHERAPY FOR AGING SKIN:

- Moisturize with essential oils such as benzoin, bergamot, chamomile, fennel, geranium, lavender, palmarosa, patchouli, sandalwood, and vetiver. You may add them to a hydrolat or mild lotion, create a massage oil by diluting a few drops with vegetable carrier oil, or make a cool compress. The best time to moisturize is when your skin is already damp or hydrated, as damp skin can retain more moisture. Be sure to moisturize your body as well as your face.

- Neroli and fennel possess rejuvenating properties similar to natural hormones. To firm and enliven sagging skin, dilute several drops of fennel with a tablespoon of carrier oil and use to massage your face and neck.

- To add moisture and reduce the appearance of wrinkles and spider veins, dilute several drops of the essential oil of carrot seed with a tablespoon of vegetable carrier oil and use a moist cotton or gauze pad to massage into skin once daily at bedtime. Alternatively apply a cool compress, or spritz affected areas with a hydrolat once a day at bedtime. Frankincense and palmarosa may also be used, but are generally not as effective as carrot seed.

- To encourage age spots to fade, dilute two or three drops of the essential oils of benzoin or lemon with a tablespoon of vegetable carrier oil and apply twice a day.

- To reduce the appearance of skin eruptions that may increase with hormonal changes during menopause, apply two or three drops of juniper, lavender, or tea tree diluted with a tablespoon of vegetable carrier oil. Use twice a day as needed. Other essential oils that may be used for this purpose include bergamot, cajeput, calendula, camphor, chamomile, cypress, eucalyptus, geranium, mint, myrrh, myrtle, neroli, palmarosa, patchouli, peppermint, rosemary, sage, thyme, and verbena.

- Circulation slows as you age, but massage with essential oils such as lavender, neroli, bergamot, and ylang-ylang can help pick up the slack. These oils naturally stimulate circulation and encourage the sloughing off of the old and the growth of new skin cells. Massage your face and body each night with several drops of one of these essential oils diluted with a tablespoon of a nourishing base oil such as apricot, avocado, evening primrose, sweet almond, or wheat germ.

ANOREXIA

Anorexia is a very serious disease in which dieting spins out of control, usually due to perceived or real social pressures to achieve "the ideal weight." People who suffer from this disease—most often teenage girls—lose all interest in food and see themselves as overweight no matter how dangerously thin they may actually become. Anorexia is a potentially fatal disease, and if you or your child suffer from anorexia, consult your physician. Supportive treatments offered by aromatherapy include the use of essential oils to reduce stress and stimulate appetite.

AROMATHERAPY FOR ANOREXIA:

- Oils that are comforting and grounding can help relieve the intense anxiety that accompanies anorexia. Try adding sandalwood, vetiver, and frankincense to massages and baths.

- Use an aroma lamp, ring, or diffuser to introduce the scents of marjoram, melissa, or thyme into your environment. These may lessen tension and spark appetite.

- To relieve stress, add several drops of one or a combination of these essential oils to your bath, or dilute with a tablespoon of vegetable carrier oil and use as a massage oil on the stomach, hands, and feet.

ANXIETY

Anxiety and tension pervade modern life and may eventually have a negative impact on your physical as well as your emotional well-being. Anxiety can impose unnecessary burdens on your heart, digestive system, immune system, and so forth. Anxiety can lead to headaches and can worsen conditions such as headaches and PMS. Aromatherapy offers various supportive strategies for anxiety, such as massages, baths, and diffusions with essential oils.

AROMATHERAPY FOR ANXIETY:

- To relieve anxiety related to panic and fear, try soothing, grounding essential oils such as vetiver, sandalwood, and frankincense. Everlasting is also grounding, but less intense. Dilute several drops of one of these essential oils with a carrier oil and massage into your upper chest, where a lot of emotional tension is often held. This will help calm you and bring you back down to earth.

• Neroli, petitgrain, and marjoram are calming to the nervous system and may be diffused into the atmosphere, mixed with a massage oil, or added to your bath to relieve anxiety. To tranquilize disturbed feelings, lie down and relax with a hot neroli, petitgrain, or marjoram compress on your abdomen.

• For depression relating to grieving or anxiety, rose otto combined with benzoin is very soothing and calming. Rose oil has been known throughout time to be healing in this way. Rose otto is the essential oil that is distilled from highly perfumed damask roses, and this is the rose oil with the greatest therapeutic value. Use in massage. A rose bath can also be very soothing, especially to those who naturally have a somewhat nervous nature.

• Disperse the soothing scent of clary sage throughout your environment to ease tension and anxiety.

ARTHRITIS

Arthritis is actually an umbrella term for more than a hundred different joint diseases, in which one or more of the joints in your body becomes swollen and inflamed. Although it is most common in older people, arthritis can strike at any age and ranges from mild aches to severe impairment.

Supportive aromatherapy treatments include compresses, massages, and baths using essential oils. The key to treating arthritis or any joint pain is to remove inflammation, so using essential oils that promote local circulation to remove toxins and swelling is important. Rosemary and juniper are the most effective essential oils for this purpose, and lavender can be added to the mix for its analgesic qualities.

AROMATHERAPY FOR ARTHRITIS:

- To relieve pain, apply a hot compress made with three drops of rosemary or juniper and two drops of lavender diluted with a tablespoon of vegetable carrier oil. With arthritis, arnica is by far the most effective carrier oil because of its own natural anti-inflammatory properties.

- Massage aching joints with a combination of these essential oils.

- Add a few diluted drops of rosemary or juniper oil to your bath. A drop or two of lavender is also soothing.

- Other essential oils that may be used in the treatment of arthritis include angelica, bay, birch, clove, eucalyptus, laurel, and pine.

ASTHMA

Asthma is a common condition (especially in children) that usually involves coughing, wheezing, and shortness of breath. If you or your child has asthma, see your doctor. Since asthma is often linked to allergies—and an essential oil may trigger an allergic reaction in a susceptible person—all supportive aromatherapy for asthma must be under the close supervision of your doctor. Eucalyptus is the most helpful essential oil in cases of asthma.

AROMATHERAPY FOR ASTHMA:

• For nighttime relief of asthma, place a bowl of hot water containing one drop of eucalyptus and three drops of benzoin at your bedside.

• Place a hot compress made with a drop of eucalyptus and four drops of benzoin diluted with a tablespoon of vegetable carrier oil on your chest. You may also add a drop or two of Roman chamomile to this mixture; Roman chamomile is antispasmodic and calming.

• Add a few drops of clary sage or melissa to your bath, or use an aroma lamp, ring, or diffuser to disperse their scents into your environment.

• Frankincense may be inhaled several times a day to slow and deepen breathing. Add two drops to a quart of hot water, cover your head with a towel, and rest

your face about twelve inches above the bowl or pot.
Breathe deeply.

ATHLETE'S FOOT

Athlete's foot is an itchy and uncomfortable fungal skin
disorder. Your doctor may prescribe antifungal medication for athlete's foot. Supportive aromatherapy for athlete's foot consists of the local application of essential
oils, especially tea tree.

AROMATHERAPY FOR ATHLETE'S FOOT:

- Apply a small amount of undiluted tea tree or lavender oil to affected areas up to three times daily.

- Spritz with a lavender hydrolat, to which you can add
  several drops of tea tree oil.

- Dilute five drops of geranium or three drops of thyme
  with a tablespoon of vegetable carrier oil. Apply twice
  a day.

Backache

Maybe you staggered home with a bag of groceries that was too heavy, or perhaps you picked it up the wrong way. (The right way is to bend your knees, lean down, and then lift.) You may suffer from chronic back problems if you have poor posture, if you lean over a computer keyboard all day at work, or if you cart your toddler around town each day. There are as many causes of back pain as there are backaches.

The most effective supportive aromatherapy for backache is massage with essential oils. Massage encourages blood flow to tired, sore, or torn muscle tissues. A helpful synergistic blend combines antispasmodic essential oils with the classic anti-inflammatory carrier oil, arnica. Essential oils may also be added to baths, or diffused into the air when backaches are stress-related. If backaches persist, see your doctor to determine and treat their underlying cause.

AROMATHERAPY FOR BACKACHE:

- Dilute five drops each of the powerful antispasmodic oils Roman chamomile and *Lavender officinalis* with the anti-inflammatory carrier oil, arnica. Add two drops of marjoram, warm the oil, and massage into the back with an upward stroke to relax.

- Relax in a hot bath with a few drops of lavender, juniper, pine, or rosemary.

• Apply a hot birch, cinnamon, or laurel compress to your back.

• Dilute any one of the essential oils mentioned here— birch, cinnamon, laurel, lavender, juniper, pine, and rosemary—with a tablespoon of vegetable carrier oil. Have your partner massage this mixture into the muscles of your back.

• Since backaches are often stress-related, you may also want to diffuse a soothing oil into the air around you. Popular stress-busters include the essential oils of Roman chamomile, clary sage, geranium, lavender, melissa, rose, and sandalwood.

BAD BREATH

Bad breath can have many causes. Illness, poor hygiene, or stress can lead to bad breath—or you may simply have eaten a garlicky meal and your date did not. If bad breath persists alongside other medical problems, you should consult a heath care professional. In the meantime creating your own mouthwashes with essential oils may solve your problem.

AROMATHERAPY FOR BAD BREATH:

• An essential oil such as tea tree, which has strong antibacterial properties, can help banish bad breath.

Add a drop of tea tree oil to a cup of water, sweeten with a drop of peppermint, and use as a mouthwash.

• Basil, bergamot, clary sage, lavender, lemon, myrrh, rose, and ylang-ylang, alone or in combination, can also be used in this way to freshen your breath.

BRONCHITIS

Bronchitis, which may be either acute or chronic, is an inflammation of the bronchi, the airways of the lungs. Bronchitis is characterized by persistent coughs that bring up phlegm. Acute bronchitis usually follows a cold or flu, whereas people who smoke or who are continually subjected to pollution are most likely to suffer from chronic bronchitis. While bronchitis requires a trip to your medical doctor, supportive aromatherapy for bronchitis includes inhaling essential oils and adding them to baths and massage oils.

AROMATHERAPY FOR BRONCHITIS:

• *Eucalyptus globulus* or *Eucalyptus radiata*—which are natural expectorants—may be inhaled several times a day to relieve the lung and sinus congestion that accompanies bronchitis. Add three drops to a quart of hot water, cover your head with a towel, and rest your face about twelve inches above the bowl or pot. Breathe deeply. A drop or two of thyme or everlasting may also be used for this purpose.

- A combination of three drops of eucalyptus or one or two drops of thyme diluted with a tablespoon of vegetable carrier oil may help ease breathing difficulties. It is also effective to add several drops of an antispasmodic such as Roman chamomile. Massage the chest with this preparation several times a day.

- Disperse eucalyptus into the air via an aroma lamp, ring, or diffuser, or add a few drops to your bath to relieve congestion.

- Eucalyptus may be combined with angelica, benzoin, or niaouli in the above remedies.

- Diluted thyme oil may be inhaled several times a day to relieve lung and sinus congestion due to bronchitis. Thyme is a natural expectorant. Add one or two drops to a quart of hot water, cover your head with a towel, and rest your face about twelve inches above the bowl or pot. Breathe deeply.

- A combination of one or two drops of thyme diluted with a tablespoon of vegetable carrier oil may also ease breathing difficulties. Massage the chest with this preparation several times a day.

- Diffuse the aromas of bergamot, cajeput, frankincense, or laurel into the air to relieve respiratory discomfort.

- A combination of several drops of niaouli or frankincense diluted with a tablespoon of vegetable carrier oil may ease breathing difficulties. Massage the chest with this preparation several times a day.

- Diffuse clary sage or niaouli into the air to relieve congestion.

- As you recover from bronchitis, diffuse the warm, stimulating, and restorative scents of bay, cinnamon, or clove into the air.

- Inhaling the steam of cypress oil may have an overall beneficial effect on the respiratory system.

- Diffuse naturally antiseptic lavender into the air for preventive maintenance.

BRUISES

When you bump your shin against the coffee table, or when your child falls on the playground, damaged blood vessels under the skin will cause a bruise to form. Bruises are also a common result of minor cosmetic surgery.

Only very serious and persistent bruises require medical attention. Cool compresses using essential oils may ease the discomfort and speed the healing of bruises.

AROMATHERAPY FOR BRUISES:

- Apply a cool compress made with several drops of calendula, cypress, everlasting, geranium, lavender, or marjoram diluted with a tablespoon of vegetable carrier oil. Use up to three times daily.

- Combine five drops of angelica with a tablespoon of carrier oil and apply three times a day. (Avoid exposure to the sun directly after use.)

- To speed healing from minor surgery, add several drops of everlasting (which breaks down scar tissue and eases discoloration) and rosemary (which stimulates local circulation) to a tablespoon of the base oil of arnica. (Because even minor surgery may lead to complications, consult your medical professional to make sure this preparation is right for you.)

BURNS

Any serious burn, in which the skin has blistered or broken, should be examined by your physician. If you burn yourself, immediately plunge the affected area in cold running water.

It was the twentieth-century founder of aromatherapy, French scientist René-Maurice Gattefossé, who discovered the therapeutic properties of essential oils when he burned himself badly in the laboratory. He plunged his hand into a beaker of lavender and within twenty minutes the heat from the burn disappeared. He observed that the wound healed much more quickly as well due to this immersion. Lavender's antiseptic and anti-inflammatory properties make it an ideal treatment for burns.

AROMATHERAPY FOR BURNS:

- For minor burns the classic remedy in aromatherapy is lavender. A few drops of undiluted lavender may speed the healing of burns. Do *not* dilute in a vegetable carrier oil, which may further aggravate a burn. Cover the burn with a loose, damp compress so that it can breathe. Be careful not to block air flow.

- A drop or two of calendula oil blended in a mild lotion may also help burns heal more quickly.

CELLULITE

Cellulite, those distinctive dimples of fat with which many of us are all too familiar, often begins to appear on the thighs and buttocks with hormonal changes as you age (especially if you are overweight). The jury is still out on whether anything can really be done to reduce cellulite, but massages and baths using essential oils may be of some help.

AROMATHERAPY FOR CELLULITE:

- A cypress, fennel, geranium, grapefruit, juniper, lavender, lemon, lime, orange, or rosemary massage may increase circulation and reduce the appearance of cellulite.

- A few drops of these essential oils in a warm bath may also be beneficial. Rub the skin first with a loofah (a rough sponge) to stimulate circulation.

COLDS

Most common colds respond to home treatments such as rest, vitamin C, and supportive aromatherapy. If a cold persists or leads to secondary infections such as bronchitis or sinusitis, you should see your doctor.

AROMATHERAPY FOR COLDS:

- *Eucalyptus globulus,* a natural expectorant, may be inhaled several times a day to improve lung and sinus congestion due to colds. Add three drops to a quart of hot water, cover your head with a towel, and rest your face about twelve inches above the bowl or pot. Breathe deeply. A drop or two of thyme or everlasting may also be used for this purpose.

- Combine several drops of eucalyptus or one or two drops of thyme with a tablespoon of vegetable carrier oil. Massage the chest with this preparation several times a day to ease breathing difficulties.

- Disperse eucalyptus into the air via an aroma lamp, ring, or diffuser, or add a few drops to your bath to relieve congestion.

- Add a few drops of peppermint oil to a bowl of hot water and breathe deeply to clear your sinuses.

- Gargle with a cup of warm water and two drops of thyme, a powerful antibacterial oil.

- Diffuse hyssop into the air or apply a hot hyssop compress to ease congestion and suppress coughs.

- Several drops of niaouli, bergamot, or frankincense diluted with a tablespoon of vegetable carrier oil may also ease breathing difficulties. Massage the chest with this preparation several times a day.

- Diffuse angelica, bergamot, cajeput, clary sage, frankincense, or niaouli into the air to relieve congestion.

- Pine may be inhaled at the first sign of a cold. Dilute five drops of the essential oil with a tablespoon of vegetable carrier oil and massage into the chest. (You may substitute cypress, eucalyptus, or hyssop for two of the pine drops for an even more effective synergistic remedy.)

- Apply a hot pine compress to the chest at the first sign of infection.

- A drop or two of the essential oil of rosemary diluted with a tablespoon of vegetable carrier oil may be applied to the chest to ease breathing problems.

- Angelica, chamomile, cinnamon, clove, juniper, lavender, lime, niaouli, pine, rosemary, and thyme are among the many essential oils that may be diffused into the air to prevent the spread of germs during cold and flu season.

- As you recover from a cold, diffuse the warm and stimulating scents of bay, cinnamon, or clove into the air. Cinnamon is particularly restorative when you are recovering from a cold.

- Inhaling the steam of cypress oil may have an overall beneficial effect on the respiratory system.

COLD SORES

A cold sore is actually herpes of the mouth. Usually it is herpes simplex. Once you have experienced cold sores, you are likely to get them again. Cold sores may be triggered by stress, your menstrual cycle, an upper respiratory infection, or overexposure to the sun.

There have been a number of studies showing the effectiveness of melissa, and many cold-sore sufferers have had success with tea tree or *Lavender officinalis* applied directly to the sores. Both are very drawing and help ease the discomfort of the itching or tingling sensation.

AROMATHERAPY FOR COLD SORES:

- Apply a drop of undiluted tea tree, lavender, calendula, or chamomile oil at the first sign of a cold sore. An itching or tingling sensation usually precedes the actual lesion.

- Apply one drop of melissa or bergamot oil diluted with a teaspoon of vegetable carrier oil at the first sign of an outbreak.

COLIC

Few remedies are safe enough for use with babies, but Roman chamomile is one of them. If your baby is crying inconsolably and you are unable to calm her, she may be suffering from colic. Walking or rocking your baby may calm her down, and you may also want to try this mild natural remedy.

AROMATHERAPY FOR COLIC:

- Combine one drop of Roman chamomile with a teaspoon of vegetable carrier oil. Massage in a clockwise direction onto your baby's tummy. Follow by placing a warm Roman-chamomile compress on the tummy.

CONJUNCTIVITIS

Conjunctivitis is a very common eye problem, in which the mucous membrane is inflamed due to a bacterial or viral infection. The eyes are usually red and irritated, and there is often a sticky discharge. Your doctor will prescribe a medication that will quickly take care of the problem, while supportive aromatherapy for conjunctivitis includes the application of cool compresses.

AROMATHERAPY FOR CONJUNCTIVITIS:

- Spritz a myrtle hydrolat onto a cotton pad and place over the eyelid. Alternatively dampen the cotton pad, add a drop of myrtle, and place on the eyelid. (Never apply this or any other essential oil directly into the eyes.)

- A cool German-chamomile compress may also help relieve the itching and discomfort of conjunctivitis.

CONSTIPATION

Occasional constipation, the inability to have a normal bowel movement, may be relieved by an essential-oil massage. You should also pay attention to your diet (are you eating enough fiber?) and lifestyle habits (are you under stress? are you getting enough exercise and rest?). Supportive aromatherapy for constipation consists of the use of the citrus oils, fennel, and rosemary. If constipation persists, see your doctor.

AROMATHERAPY FOR CONSTIPATION:

- The citrus oils, especially orange (*Citrus aurantium*), are an effective treatment for constipation. Gently massage several drops diluted with a tablespoon of vegetable carrier oil in a clockwise direction around the abdomen. Using fingertips, begin just below the right lower rib, trace beneath the rib up to the sternum, and continue down the left rib cage to just above the groin. This will stimulate peristalsis.

- Fennel oil is also very balancing for digestive problems.

- Massage your stomach with several drops of rosemary diluted with a tablespoon of vegetable carrier oil.

COUGHS

Coughing accompanies a number of respiratory ailments, such as colds and bronchitis. If your cough is persistent or is accompanied by other symptoms, such as a high fever or muscle aches and pains, you may want to see your doctor. Supportive aromatherapy for coughs consists of massages, compresses, and diffusions of essential oils.

AROMATHERAPY FOR COUGHS:

- Eucalyptus may be inhaled several times a day to improve lung and sinus congestion due to coughs, as it is a natural expectorant. Add three drops to a quart of hot water, cover your head with a towel, and rest your face about twelve inches above the bowl or pot.

Breathe deeply. One or two drops of thyme or everlasting may also be used in this way.

- Dilute several drops of eucalyptus or one or two drops of thyme with a tablespoon of vegetable carrier oil to help ease breathing difficulties. Combine with an antispasmodic such as *Lavender officinalis.* Massage the chest with this preparation several times a day.

- Disperse eucalyptus into the air via an aroma lamp, ring, or diffuser, or add a few drops to your bath to relieve congestion.

- Eucalyptus may be combined with angelica or benzoin in the above remedies.

- Diffuse hyssop into the air or apply a hot hyssop compress to ease congestion and suppress coughs.

- Several drops of niaouli or frankincense diluted with a tablespoon of vegetable carrier oil may also ease breathing difficulties. Massage the chest with this preparation several times a day.

- Diffuse niaouli, cajeput, or frankincense into the air to relieve congestion.

- As you recover, use an aroma lamp to diffuse the warm, stimulating, and restorative scents of bay, cinnamon, or clove into the air.

- Inhaling the steam of cypress oil may have a beneficial effect on the respiratory system.

DANDRUFF

Excess dandruff is usually due to dry skin, overuse of hair care products, stress, or illness. Before you turn to very strong dandruff shampoos, which can be excessively drying to the scalp, you may want to try aromatherapy.

AROMATHERAPY FOR DANDRUFF:

• Rosemary increases local circulation and is stimulating to the scalp. Dilute several drops in a nutritive carrier oil such as jojoba or camellia to ease flaking.

• Other helpful oils include benzoin, cade, cedar, cypress, eucalyptus, patchouli, sage, and thyme. Try adding a drop of one of these to a mild shampoo.

• Pretreat your scalp to a massage with a small amount of a diluted essential oil. Then wrap a warm towel around your head for two hours (or overnight) before shampooing.

DEPRESSION

Depression may be due to a lack of stimulation, or an overabundance of stimulation. Accordingly you may use stimulating or calming essential oils to help relieve depression. All the citrus oils are wonderful antidepressants, especially in the wintertime. If depression persists, you should see your doctor.

STIMULATING AROMATHERAPY FOR DEPRESSION:

- Citrus oils (grapefruit, lemon, lime, neroli, orange, tangerine, verbena, etc.) are very uplifting and balancing to the nervous system. They can provide a welcome break when you are feeling overwhelmed by life. Diffuse them into the air or mix with a massage oil or mild lotion. You may also dilute them in a carrier oil (citrus oils alone will irritate the skin) and add to your bath.

- Orange and tangerine are fresh and lively scents that add good cheer and are considered especially appropriate for children.

- Disperse rosemary into the air around you or add a few drops to your bath to give your spirits a lift.

RELAXING AROMATHERAPY FOR DEPRESSION:

- Neroli, petitgrain, and marjoram are calming to the nervous system and may be diffused into the atmosphere, mixed with a massage oil, or added to your bath to relieve depression. To tranquilize disturbed feelings, lie down and relax with a hot neroli, petitgrain, or marjoram compress on your abdomen.

- For depression relating to grieving or anxiety, rose otto combined with benzoin is very soothing and calming. Rose oil has been known throughout time to be healing in this way. Rose otto is the essential oil that is distilled from highly perfumed damask roses, and this is the rose oil with the greatest therapeutic value. Use in massage or take rose baths, which can be very soothing, especially to those who naturally have a somewhat nervous nature.

• To relieve anxiety, panic, and fear, turn to calming and grounding essential oils such as vetiver, sandalwood, and frankincense. Dilute with a carrier oil and massage into the upper chest, where a great deal of emotional tension is hidden. Grounding oils are calming and can help bring you back down to earth.

• Disperse the soothing scent of clary sage throughout your environment to ease tension and anxiety.

• Circulate the fresh scent of myrtle through the air via an aroma lamp, ring, or diffuser to cleanse the mind and spirit and strengthen focus. This is particularly helpful during meditation.

• The warming and relaxing aroma of jasmine may be diffused into the atmosphere to relieve depression, low self-confidence, and sexual tension. You may also add a few drops to your bath or dilute with a tablespoon of vegetable carrier oil and, using gentle circular motions, massage into your abdomen, lower back, temples, and neck.

Detoxification

Detoxification—an elaborate term for your body's natural way of eliminating toxins—is a process that strengthens your immune system. The immune system is your body's network of natural defensive resources. In recent years our immune systems have been battered with a daily dose of hundreds of toxins: pollutants in the air we breathe, additives in processed foods, chemicals in tap water, and hormones and pesticides in fresh meat and fruits. The residues of common substances such as household cleaners, paint, and cosmetics also need to be broken down and eliminated by your body, as do tobacco, alcohol, and caffeine.

To enable your body to break down toxins quickly and efficiently, you can help by maintaining your own health through a balanced diet and exercise program. You can also avoid negative habits that overburden the immune system, such as smoking and drug use. Supportive aromatherapy for detoxification includes the use of essential oils to improve blood circulation and lymphatic flow. For example, when you massage your body with oils such as rosemary and juniper, you tone the lymph glands and speed the elimination of toxins from your body.

AROMATHERAPY FOR DETOXIFICATION:

- A juniper bath is an invaluable aid for detoxification. Dilute several drops of the essential oil with a tablespoon of vegetable carrier oil and add to warm bath-water. Everlasting may be substituted for juniper.

• Juniper may also be diffused into the air via an aroma lamp, ring, or diffuser to detoxify the environment and prevent the spread of germs in enclosed spaces.

• Add a few drops of rosemary to your bath to stimulate the elimination of toxins through your skin.

• Diffuse lavender, a natural antiseptic, into the environment to help prevent the spread of germs in enclosed spaces. At home use an aroma lamp, ring, or diffuser. In cars or airplanes, where air is constantly recirculated, spritz yourself with a lavender hydrolat, or moisten a tissue or handkerchief with a drop or two of lavender oil and simply keep it close at hand.

• Pine may be circulated through the air via an aroma lamp, ring, or diffuser to prevent the spread of germs, and get rid of smoke and other heavy odors.

• Add a drop of an essential oil to a cup of water and throw on the rocks in your sauna. This will stimulate the release of toxins from your skin. Good choices include rosemary, pine, cypress, birch, lavender, bergamot, niaouli, lemon, and lime.

DIARRHEA

Diarrhea, an increase in the frequency and fluidity of your bowel movements, may be acute or chronic. Acute diarrhea may be simply a case of spicy or fatty food that didn't sit right with you—but if it is severe and lasts longer than twenty-four hours, you should see your doctor. You may be suffering from a case of food poisoning.

Chronic diarrhea may be a symptom of a more critical underlying disorder, such as ulcerative colitis or Crohn's disease. Since diarrhea can lead to serious dehydration and depletion of your body's supply of potassium, it should not be treated lightly. See your doctor.

In mild, passing cases of diarrhea, especially when diarrhea is brought on by stress, aromatherapy offers supportive remedies such as hot compresses, baths, massages, and diffusions of essential oils.

AROMATHERAPY FOR DIARRHEA:

- Roman chamomile is a helpful treatment for diarrhea, especially when it is stress-related. Dilute a few drops of chamomile with a tablespoon of vegetable carrier oil and massage into the abdomen, using broad, circular strokes. You can also make a hot chamomile compress and rest with it on your tummy, or add a few drops of the essential oil to your bath.

- A hot cajeput, laurel, marjoram, or thyme compress on the abdomen may provide comfort during an episode of diarrhea.

- Diffuse the essential oil of peppermint into the air to help relieve the nausea that often accompanies diarrhea.

- Fennel oil is also very balancing for digestive problems.

EARACHES

Earaches often follow a cold or flu, especially in children. Many ear infections are bacterial and require a visit to your doctor. Supportive aromatherapy involves the use of essential oils to relieve earache pain.

AROMATHERAPY FOR EARACHES:

- To relieve a painful earache, dip a cotton swab in calendula oil and place the oil in the ear overnight.

- You may also dilute a drop of chamomile or marjoram with a teaspoon of vegetable carrier oil, dip a cotton swab in this mixture, and place in the ear overnight.

Eczema

Eczema is a general term for any noncontagious, inflammatory skin rash. Many people who have allergies also have eczema, which can be excruciatingly itchy and uncomfortable. Supportive aromatherapy involves the use of essential oils to soothe the itching and burning of eczema.

AROMATHERAPY FOR ECZEMA:

- One of the best treatments for eczema is German chamomile. Its primary chemical constituent is azulene, an anti-inflammatory agent. Dilute one to two drops of German chamomile with a tablespoon of the carrier oil calendula and apply to the affected areas.

- Dilute several drops of bergamot, birch, cade, cajeput, everlasting, geranium, juniper, lavender, myrrh, patchouli, or yarrow with a tablespoon of vegetable carrier oil, and apply to the affected areas twice a day.

- Take a sponge bath using several drops of lemon or orange oil diluted with a quart of water.

- Add a few drops of rosemary oil to your daily bath.

- Apply a cool rose compress to affected areas.

EYE INFLAMMATION

Puffy eyes is a condition that becomes more common as you age, and may be a result of too much work, too little sleep, overexposure to the sun, or an excess of emotional or mental stress. Bathing the eyes in ice-cold water is often helpful, while the best supportive aromatherapy for eye inflammation is the application of soothing cool compresses over the eyelids. Essential oils should *never* be placed directly in the eyes.

AROMATHERAPY FOR EYE INFLAMMATION:

- Apply a cool German-chamomile compress. Steeped teabags cooled in the refrigerator will do the trick.

- A cool myrtle, rose, or marigold compress may also help relieve swollen, tired eyes.

FATIGUE

Fatigue may come from two sources: You may be exhausted and require a stimulating essential oil to give you a pick-me-up, or you may be suffering from nervous tension and stress, in which case a calming essential oil will do the trick. The best way to prevent fatigue is to lead a healthy lifestyle, incorporating a healthy diet and a good balance of rest and exercise.

STIMULATING AROMATHERAPY FOR FATIGUE:

- One of the best oils to combat mental fatigue is basil, a stimulating oil that aids concentration. Try diffusing basil into your environment while finishing a report or studying for exams.

- Because of its uplifting qualities, rosemary may be diffused into the atmosphere to relieve mental and physical fatigue. You may also add rosemary to your morning bath if you are overtired and need an extra boost of energy to face the day ahead.

- A few drops of eucalyptus may be diffused through the air or added to a bath or massage oil to relieve mental and physical fatigue.

- Grapefruit and petitgrain may be diffused into the air, mixed with a massage oil or mild lotion, or added to your bath to combat fatigue.

- Juniper and lime are stimulating scents that may be dispersed into your environment to relieve exhaustion and restore energy and strength.

- Diffuse lemongrass into the air around you or add a few drops to your bath to relieve fatigue and increase concentration.

- The pungent aroma of several drops of celery oil in your bath can act as a pick-me-up after a long day at the office.

- Diffuse the essential oil of verbena into your environment to counteract the effects of daily tiredness and depression.

RELAXING AROMATHERAPY FOR FATIGUE:

- Nothing beats lavender for relieving stress-induced fatigue. It is calming to the central nervous system, and studies have shown its effectiveness in treating insomnia. Keep a lavender hydrolat close at hand and treat yourself to an occasional spray. You may also diffuse the scent of lavender through your room via an aroma lamp, or try sprinkling a few drops on the pillow at night before bed.

- Geranium has a relaxing, flowery scent that may be diffused into the atmosphere or added to your bath to relieve fatigue. You may also dilute several drops of geranium with a tablespoon of vegetable carrier oil and massage into your neck and temples or stomach.

- The calming essential oil of clary sage may be circulated through the air via an aroma lamp, ring, or diffuser to reduce nervous tension and fatigue.

FEVER

Fever is a sign that your body is fighting an infection. It's important to detect and treat the underlying cause of a fever. In the meantime aromatherapy can help you feel better and bring the fever down.

AROMATHERAPY FOR FEVER:

- A lukewarm bath with lavender or peppermint may have a cooling effect on feverish conditions.

- A cold eucalyptus compress applied to the legs or feet can help bring down a fever.

- To relieve aching muscles that often accompany fevers, dilute five drops of palmarosa with a tablespoon of vegetable carrier oil and massage into the chest, shoulders, and neck.

FLATULENCE

(*Gas*)

Gas is formed in the stomach and intestines through poor diet or swallowed air and is dispelled through the anus. Aromatherapy offers help in avoiding this embarrassing and uncomfortable condition.

AROMATHERAPY FOR FLATULENCE:

- A hot marjoram compress on the abdomen may provide comfort during episodes of flatulence.

- Diffuse the essential oil of peppermint into the air to help relieve nausea and gas.

- A warm compress of fennel is often an effective remedy for gas resulting from indigestion.

FLU

The flu, or influenza, is a viral infection that involves respiratory discomfort, muscle aches and pains, headache, fever, and chills. The flu can cause great discomfort, and may be dangerous for the very young, the elderly, and those whose immune systems have already been compromised by other diseases.

If you think you have the flu, you should see your doctor. Supportive aromatherapy for flu discomfort includes hot compresses, massages, and diffusions of essential oils. Essential oils are rapidly absorbed into the skin; commercially this has been put to good effect with eucalyptus, one of the main ingredients in Vicks VapoRub.

AROMATHERAPY FOR THE FLU:

- *Eucalyptus globulus* may be inhaled several times a day to improve lung and sinus congestion. Add three drops to a quart of hot water, cover your head with a towel, and rest your face about twelve inches above the bowl or pot. Breathe deeply. A drop or two of thyme or everlasting may also be used for this purpose.

- Combine several drops of eucalyptus or one or two drops of thyme with a tablespoon of vegetable carrier oil. Massage the chest with this preparation several times a day to ease breathing difficulties.

- Diffuse eucalyptus into the air or add a few drops to your bath to relieve congestion.

- Diffuse the warm aroma of laurel into the air to relieve the discomfort of flu symptoms. Laurel, like eucalyptus, is a natural expectorant.

- A combination of several drops of angelica, frankincense, or niaouli diluted with a tablespoon of vegetable carrier oil may also ease breathing difficulties. Massage the chest with this preparation several times a day.

- Diffuse niaouli, cajeput, or frankincense into the air to relieve congestion.

- Add a few drops of peppermint oil to a bowl of hot water and breathe deeply to clear your sinuses.

- To relieve aching muscles that often accompany the flu, dilute five drops of palmarosa with a tablespoon of vegetable carrier oil and massage into the chest, shoulders, and neck.

- Pine may be inhaled at the first sign of a cold or flu. Dilute five drops of the essential oil with a tablespoon of vegetable carrier oil and massage into the chest.

(You may substitute cypress, eucalyptus, or hyssop for two of the pine drops for an even more effective synergistic remedy.)

• Apply a hot pine compress to the chest at the first sign of infection.

• A drop or two of the essential oil of rosemary diluted with a tablespoon of vegetable carrier oil may be applied to the chest to ease breathing problems.

• Angelica, chamomile, cinnamon, clove, juniper, lavender, lime, niaouli, pine, rosemary, and thyme are among the many essential oils that may be diffused into the air to prevent the spread of germs during flu season.

• As you recover from the flu, diffuse the warm, stimulating, and restorative scents of bay, cinnamon, or clove into the air.

• Inhaling the steam of cypress oil may have a beneficial effect on the respiratory system.

FOOT CARE

Our feet are among the most neglected areas of our bodies, as we subject them to serious wear and tear on a daily basis. Your feet should be moisturized on a regular basis, and a foot massage or soak can be extremely soothing. Reflexology tells us that there are over seven thousand nerve endings on each foot—so what could be better than a foot massage after a long day at the office? Foot baths are another way to soothe tired feet. Essential oils such as cypress, juniper, lavender, peppermint, rosemary, and tea tree are all helpful for foot care.

AROMATHERAPY FOR FOOT CARE:

• Massage tired, painful feet with several drops of the essential oil of your choice diluted with a tablespoon of vegetable carrier oil.

• For a relaxing foot bath, add three to five drops of an essential oil to a bowl of lukewarm water. (For a synergistic effect, choose three oils and add one drop of each.) Add a tablespoon of Epsom salts. Soak your feet for five to fifteen minutes. Cypress and tea tree, natural deodorants, are particularly helpful for those who suffer from foot odor.

• Soak swollen feet in a bowl of ice water with three drops of lavender oil. A ten-minute foot bath in cold water is refreshing and stimulates circulation.

Gum Problems

Gum disease, or pyorrhea, occupies dentists today as much as tooth decay. It begins when bacteria causes plaque to form on teeth; if the plaque is not removed, gums become inflamed and the plaque hardens into tartar. Eventually tooth loss can result. There is no substitute for good dental hygiene, but supportive aromatherapy includes the use of various rinses with essential oils.

AROMATHERAPY FOR GUM PROBLEMS:

- Gargle with a drop of clove and two drops of thyme in a cup of warm water. (Do not swallow.)

- A drop of cypress, myrrh, lavender, rose, or tea tree may also be added to a cup of warm water to use as a mouthwash for gum problems.

HAIR CARE

Healthy, shining hair is usually the reflection of a well-balanced lifestyle. Oily hair is often due to overactive sebaceous glands or ill health, while dry and brittle hair can be a sign of poor diet, overexposure to the sun and chlorine, or excessive coloring and perming.

One of the most valuable essential oils in hair care is lavender, which naturally balances sebum production. When sebaceous glands produce excess sebum, you have oily hair; when there is not enough sebum, hair becomes dry and dull. Many essential oils can be used to help keep your hair healthy, and to deal with hair problems as they arise.

AROMATHERAPY FOR NORMAL HAIR:

- Normal hair, which is neither dry nor oily, benefits from regular shampooing with a mild shampoo to which you may add a drop of one of these nourishing essential oils: lavender, geranium, carrot seed, lemon, or rosemary.

- Create your own personalized conditioner by adding a drop of the essential oil of carrot seed or geranium to a regular mild conditioner for normal hair. Apply generously once or twice a week after shampooing. Leave on for ten minutes and then rinse well.

AROMATHERAPY FOR DRY HAIR:

- Moisturizing essential oils for dry hair include lavender, birch, carrot seed, geranium, parsley, sandalwood, and yarrow. Try adding a drop to your regular mild shampoo and use several times a week.

- To condition dry hair, combine a drop or two of these essential oils with a tablespoon of a rich base oil, such as sweet almond, avocado, borage, jojoba, or sesame. Once a week pretreat your scalp with a massage using this mixture. Then wrap a warm towel around your head for two hours (or overnight) before rinsing well with a mild shampoo. If you have fair hair, you can finish up by rinsing with the juice of a freshly squeezed lemon; you can cap off dark hair by rinsing with two ounces of cider vinegar. These will give your hair extra shine and greater manageability.

AROMATHERAPY FOR OILY HAIR:

• Shampoo daily with a mild shampoo to which you have added a drop of rosemary, lavender, eucalyptus, cypress, or lemon. While these are the best essential oils for oily hair, basil, sage, thyme, and yarrow may also be helpful.

• On a weekly basis dilute a drop or two of one of these essential oils with a tablespoon of a nourishing base oil such as jojoba or camellia. Pretreat your scalp with a massage using this mixture. Then wrap a warm towel around your head for two hours (or overnight) before rinsing well with a mild shampoo.

AROMATHERAPY FOR DAMAGED OR CHEMICALLY TREATED HAIR:

• Helpful essential oils for permed, colored, or damaged hair are cade and German chamomile. Try adding a drop to your regular mild shampoo and use several times a week.

• To condition damaged or chemically treated hair, combine two or three drops of cade or German chamomile with a tablespoon of a rich base oil such as jojoba or sesame. Once a week pretreat your scalp to a massage with this mixture. Then wrap a warm towel around your head for two hours (or overnight) before rinsing well with a mild shampoo.

AROMATHERAPY FOR HAIR COLOR:

• To help condition dry dark hair and keep it shiny, add a drop of patchouli and a drop of ylang-ylang to a tablespoon of vegetable carrier oil and massage into your scalp. Then wrap a warm towel around your head for an hour before rinsing well with a mild shampoo.

• Brunettes can also add a drop of rosemary to their shampoo to give it an added shine, while blondes can liven up their hair color with lemon or German chamomile.

HAIR LOSS

Women as well as men experience a natural thinning of hair with age, and hair loss can also be due to illness, stress, or overuse of perms, dryers, or hot curlers. Medical reasons for hair loss should be ruled out by your doctor. In the meantime essential oils can help increase local circulation and stimulate hair follicles in the scalp.

AROMATHERAPY FOR HAIR LOSS:

• Stimulating rosemary increases local circulation and acts as a tonic to encourage hair growth. Dilute several drops in a nutritive carrier oil such as jojoba or camellia and massage into the scalp.

• Add a few drops of essential oils such as bay, birch, cade, laurel, or yarrow to your regular mild shampoo to encourage hair growth.

- Pretreat your scalp to a massage with a small, diluted amount of one of the above oils. Then wrap a warm towel around your head for two hours (or overnight) before shampooing.

HANGOVER

Most of us have occasionally overindulged at a wedding or office party, only to pay the price the next morning. A hangover generally involves a throbbing head, dehydration, nausea, and an overall resolution never to feel this way again. A number of essential oils can help you get back to feeling like your normal self again.

AROMATHERAPY FOR HANGOVERS:

- Add a few drops of fennel, peppermint, or rose to your morning bath to relieve the nausea and discomfort of a hangover. Peppermint is an especially effective antinausea remedy.

- Apply a cool geranium or lavender compress to your forehead and neck.

- Treat yourself to a soothing spray of a lavender hydrolat.

HEADACHE

Headaches can be brought on by any number of conditions, such as tension, stress, overwork, fatigue, poor diet, overexposure to heat, or alcohol. Researchers at the neurological clinic at Universität Christin Albrechts in Kiel, Germany, recently evaluated the effectiveness of using ten grams of peppermint with a trace of eucalyptus to treat headache pain. The application of this combination to the temples and the back of the head was found to significantly reduce pain and enhance relaxation.

If headaches persist, it's important to detect and eliminate their underlying cause. Supportive aromatherapy for headaches consists of massage with essential oils.

AROMATHERAPY FOR HEADACHES:

- Roman chamomile is helpful in treating stress-related sinus headaches and migraines. Use your fingertips to lightly massage the diluted oil into the temples and sinus areas.

- Water infused with lavender can be gently massaged into the temples, the base of the skull, and around the hairline to soothe headache pain.

- A drop of basil oil diluted with a tablespoon of vegetable carrier oil can be massaged into the temples to soothe a headache.

- A massage oil containing rosemary may be gently rubbed into the temples to relieve headaches, especially migraines.

HEMORRHOIDS

Hemorrhoids are swollen varicose veins in the rectal area. Often they are due to weight gain, constipation, or pregnancy and can be controlled by following a diet high in fiber and getting plenty of exercise. Supportive aromatherapy for hemorrhoids includes the use of essential oils in warm compresses and sitzbaths. If hemorrhoids are painful or bleed, you should consult a medical professional.

AROMATHERAPY FOR HEMORRHOIDS:

- Cypress is one of the best essential oils for hemorrhoids. Add several drops to your bath, or apply a warm cypress compress.

- Dilute several drops of the essential oils of cypress, geranium, or myrtle with a tablespoon of vegetable carrier oil and gently apply once daily.

- To relieve itching, prepare a warm sitzbath with one drop of tea tree and one drop of rose in a bowl of warm water. Use once a day.

- Prepare a soothing sitzbath by diluting three drops of yarrow oil with two cups of rosewater.

HERPES SIMPLEX

Herpes is a virus that can appear as cold sores in the mouth area or as genital lesions. Once you have experienced the virus, it is in your system and may periodically reappear. A recurrence of herpes can be triggered by stress, menstrual cycles, an upper respiratory infection, or overexposure to the sun. While nothing can completely prevent or cure herpes, aromatherapy offers various supportive treatments.

AROMATHERAPY FOR HERPES SIMPLEX:

- Apply a drop of undiluted (neat) lavender or tea tree oil at the first sign of herpes. An itching or tingling sensation usually precedes the actual lesion.

- Apply one drop of melissa or bergamot oil diluted with a teaspoon of vegetable carrier oil to a cold sore or other herpes lesion at the first sign of outbreak. Again, an itching or tingling sensation signals the occurrence.

- Apply a drop of undiluted calendula or German chamomile oil to the site when you suspect an outbreak.

- To ease the pain of genital herpes, dilute several drops of rose with a tablespoon of vegetable carrier oil and dab onto the affected area.

HIGH BLOOD PRESSURE
(*Hypertension*)

If you suffer from high blood pressure, you should be under the care of a medical doctor. However, aromatherapy offers supportive remedies that can help you lower the stress that in many cases is linked to this health problem.

Lavender, bergamot, chamomile, clary sage, geranium, marjoram, melissa, orange, rose, sandalwood, and ylang-ylang are popular stress busters in aromatherapy. Try one or more of these when you encounter tension at work or home.

Another way to reduce stress is through meditation. Benzoin, cedar, frankincense, myrrh, and sandalwood are very grounding essential oils that can help you maintain focus during exercises such as yoga and meditation.

AROMATHERAPY FOR HIGH BLOOD PRESSURE (HYPERTENSION):

- Massage therapy is one of the most effective ways of normalizing blood pressure. Try a full body massage with *Lavender officinalis,* which is especially calming to the central nervous system. You may also keep a lavender hydrolat in your purse or office drawer and give yourself a calming spritz when the stress is getting to you.

- Dilute several drops of one of the other calming essential oils mentioned above with a tablespoon of vegetable carrier oil or a mild lotion and massage into the body.

- Diffuse one or more essential oils into the environment to release tension and anxiety and support calm and meditation.

- Create a soothing aromatic bath using a few drops of your favorite essential oil.

IMMUNE ENHANCEMENT

See **Detoxification.**

INDIGESTION

Indigestion is an umbrella term for a number of problems, such as diarrhea, flatulence, heartburn, nausea, and stomachaches. Indigestion may be a sign of poor diet, inadequate exercise and rest, or stress. Pregnant women often experience some temporary form of indigestion, and sometimes indigestion simply means that you ate something that did not "agree" with you. If indigestion becomes a chronic problem, you should see your doctor to rule out any serious underlying health problems. Supportive aromatherapy for indigestion includes hot compresses, massages, and diffusions of essential oils.

AROMATHERAPY FOR INDIGESTION:

- Place a hot Roman-chamomile or cajeput compress on your stomach.

- To stimulate digestion, massage your liver and stomach area with several drops of the essential oils of fennel, rosemary, or Roman chamomile diluted with a tablespoon of vegetable carrier oil. Fennel is especially helpful in this case.

- Diffuse the essential oil of peppermint into the air to help relieve indigestion, especially when it is related to nausea.

INSECT BITES AND STINGS

Insect bites and bee stings can be quite painful, but most respond well to timely home treatment with naturally antiseptic essential oils.

AROMATHERAPY FOR INSECT BITES AND STINGS:

- Apply a drop of neat (undiluted) lavender on bites and stings to relieve pain and swelling.

- A cool basil, chamomile, cinnamon, citronella, geranium, lemon, melissa, tea tree, or thyme compress may be applied to soothe the pain and itching of insect bites or bee stings.

- Apply a mixture of eight drops of myrtle diluted with a tablespoon of vegetable carrier oil.

INSECT REPELLENTS

There are a number of essential oils that act as natural insect deterrents and may prevent bites and stings by keeping pesky insects at bay. Citronella and lemongrass are popular preventive choices, while lavender is especially helpful in keeping pesky mosquitoes at bay. Other choices include basil, cajeput, cedar, cinnamon, clove, eucalyptus, fennel, geranium, juniper, myrtle, niaouli, patchouli, pine, thyme, and vetiver.

AROMATHERAPY FOR INSECT REPELLENTS:

- Citronella candles are commercially available, while any of the aromas mentioned above may be diffused into the air via aroma lamps or rings.

- When traveling, add a few drops of one of the above-mentioned essential oils to a cup of hot water. Hot water will release the scent into the air and discourage pesky guests. Place at the window or by your bed.

- Add two drops of an essential oil to your massage oil, skin lotion, or cream.

INSOMNIA

Insomnia, or an inability to sleep, is most often due to stress or anxiety. If you're tossing and turning and can't get a good night's sleep, aromatherapy offers safe and natural essential oils to relax you.

AROMATHERAPY FOR INSOMNIA:

- The essential oil of lavender (especially *Lavender officinalis*) may be diffused into the air alone or with neroli or rose to restore a sense of calm and help you get a good night's sleep.

- A lavender, marjoram, neroli, or petitgrain bath can provide comfort and relief after any stressful experience and is especially useful if you suffer from chronic anxiety or high blood pressure.

- The scents of bergamot and marjoram are balancing and relaxing. They may be diffused into the air, mixed with a massage oil, or added to your bath to promote calm and stability.

- A sweet tangerine scent may be circulated through the air via an aroma lamp, ring, or diffuser to dispel sadness and irritability and help you get a good night's sleep.

- Add a drop of lavender, neroli, rose, bergamot, orange, marjoram, or tangerine to a tissue or handkerchief by your bedside, or to the edge of your pillow, to quiet the nervous anxiety that often leads to insomnia.

JET LAG

If you've ever taken a long flight, you already know the meaning of jet lag. Fatigue, insomnia, disorientation, and muscle aches and pains number among the unpleasant consequences of jet lag. Aromatherapy offers a number of safe and natural solutions to these problems.

AROMATHERAPY FOR JET LAG:

- Spritzing with a hydrolat during a flight is a terrific way to keep skin moisturized and feel refreshed overall. The antiseptic and calming qualities of lavender water are perfect for long flights, when air is constantly recirculated.

- Place a few drops of basil to stimulate concentration—or lavender to instill calm—on a handkerchief or tissue during flight. Inhale as needed.

- If you arrive at your destination and it's already time for your first business meeting, take a quick bath or indulge in a massage with stimulating essential oils such as basil, lemongrass, peppermint, or rosemary. These oils can help you beat mental and physical fatigue.

- You may also try diffusing several drops of basil or cardamom into the air to lift your spirits and stimulate memory and concentration.

- If you're wound up and disoriented after a long trip and find it hard to get to sleep, add a few drops of lavender and ylang-ylang oils to your evening bath.

- Bergamot and marjoram are also calming and balancing fragrances that may be diffused into the air, mixed with a massage oil, or added to your bath to restore calm and stability.

MENOPAUSAL SYMPTOMS

Menopause is a natural physical transition that all women experience with age. Yet each woman's menopause is unique. Some women have few problems with menopause, while others experience symptoms such as hot flashes, sleep disturbances, mood swings, water buildup, irritability, and skin changes. Supportive aromatherapy for menopause includes the use of compresses, massages, baths, and diffusions of essential oils. Clary sage is one of the most helpful essential oils to use during menopause.

AROMATHERAPY FOR MENOPAUSAL SYMPTOMS:

- For hot flashes, apply a cold compress of clary sage. To make the compress, dip a cotton towel or washcloth into a bowl of cold water with four to six drops of the essential oil. If clary sage is not available, lavender, lemon, or melissa may be used.

- To relieve the water buildup and irritability that often accompany menopause, use circular motions to massage the diluted essential oils of clary sage, Roman chamomile, or cardamom into the stomach and lower back.

- The scents of cypress, rose, and marjoram are soothing aromas that may be diffused into the air, mixed with a massage oil, or added to your bath to counteract the mood swings and nervous tension associated with menopause.

- The restorative qualities of basil oil may help regulate periods as you approach menopause. Try rubbing a massage oil containing basil in circles around the stomach area.

- To keep your changing life in balance, add one drop of vetiver to your bath or disperse its scent into the air via an aroma lamp, ring, or diffuser.

- Lavender, bergamot, and yarrow are very calming and may be diffused into the air, mixed with a massage oil, or added to your bath to counteract sleep disturbances and stabilize mood swings.

- To encourage brown age spots to fade, dilute two or three drops of benzoin or lemon with a tablespoon of vegetable carrier oil and apply twice a day.

Also see **Aging Skin.**

MENSTRUAL DISCOMFORT

Menstrual cramps are caused by contractions of the uterus, and range from mild to debilitating. Cramps—and the depression and irritability that sometimes accompany them—are simply a fact of life for many women during their reproductive years, but aromatherapy offers many supportive remedies that you can use to cope with menstrual discomfort.

AROMATHERAPY FOR MENSTRUAL DISCOMFORT:

- Clary sage is the classic remedy for menstrual discomfort. Add a few drops to your bath or dilute several drops of the essential oil with a tablespoon of vegetable carrier oil, and, using gentle circular motions, massage into your abdomen and lower back. The essential oil of clary sage may also be circulated through the air via an aroma lamp, ring, or diffuser to reduce stress, banish moodiness, and give a general lift to your spirits.

- Lavender is very calming and may be inhaled to balance mood swings and promote stability.

- Try massage oils containing angelica, everlasting, lavender, lemon, or rose oil.

- Place a warm Roman-chamomile or yarrow compress on your stomach.

- Basil oil may help restore regular periods. Try rubbing a massage oil containing basil in circles around the stomach area.

MIGRAINE

A migraine is an especially severe recurrent headache, which is often accompanied by nausea and vomiting. Researchers have identified red wine, chocolate, and aged cheese as possible triggers of migraine headaches. If you experience periodic migraines, you should see your doctor. Supportive aromatherapy for migraines includes the use of compresses and massages with essential oils.

AROMATHERAPY FOR MIGRAINES:

- A drop of basil oil diluted with a tablespoon of vegetable carrier oil may be gently rubbed into the temples to soothe a migraine.

- Water infused with lavender can be gently massaged into the temples and neck to alleviate migraine pain. Slowly circle your temples with your fingertips.

- Chamomile is also helpful in treating stress-related migraines. Use your fingertips to lightly massage the diluted oil into the temples.

- Combine chamomile, clary sage, and lavender on a cool compress, and apply to the forehead, neck, and back of the head to ease migraine pain and discomfort.

- Diluted rosemary oil may be gently rubbed into the temples to relieve all headaches, especially migraines.

- Mix a few drops of rose, melissa, or marjoram in a tablespoon of vegetable carrier oil and gently rub into the temples to soothe a migraine.

- Massage stimulating diluted peppermint into the temples and back of the neck.

MORNING SICKNESS

Morning sickness is actually a misnomer, since this nauseous feeling can overtake you at any time during pregnancy, especially during the first trimester. While the aroma of natural essential oils may relieve morning sickness, it's best to consult your health care professional before using any remedy during pregnancy.

Peppermint is generally considered the best supportive aromatherapy for morning sickness. Some women find it helpful to rotate the essential oils they use so that a negative association does not develop between the nausea and a particular aroma. Lavender, petitgrain, and lemon are good alternatives.

AROMATHERAPY FOR MORNING SICKNESS:

- Place several drops of peppermint on your handkerchief or tissue and keep near you in your pocket or purse to inhale as needed. Alternate with lavender, petitgrain, and lemon as needed.

- Circulate the essential oil of peppermint through the air via an aroma lamp, ring, or diffuser.

- Add a drop of peppermint oil to your bath.

- Rub your abdomen with a massage oil containing peppermint.

MOTION SICKNESS

Motion sickness can overtake you (or often your child) in a car, plane, or train. The natural fragrance of the essential oil of peppermint can help relieve the nausea of motion sickness.

AROMATHERAPY FOR MOTION SICKNESS:

• Carry a small bottle of peppermint oil when you travel if you or your child are prone to motion sickness. A sniff of peppermint (from the bottle, or on a tissue or handkerchief for your child) may prevent or cure nausea and discomfort.

MUSCLE ACHES AND PAINS

Muscle aches and pains are due to a variety of causes. They may accompany illnesses such as the flu, or be a result of too little, too much, or excessively repetitive exercise. When athletes overextend themselves, their muscles can go into spasm.

Supportive aromatherapy for muscle problems includes massages, hot compresses, and baths using essential oils. Rosemary is one of the most useful essential oils for muscle aches and pains.

AROMATHERAPY FOR MUSCLE ACHES AND PAINS:

- Create a massage oil containing several drops of rosemary diluted with a tablespoon of carrier oil. With muscle aches and pains, arnica is by far the most effective carrier oil because of its own natural anti-inflammatory properties. Rub this mixture into sore muscles to increase local circulation and help remove lactic acid and cellular waste products. Birch, cajeput, fennel, and pine may be used in place of rosemary.

- A hot rosemary, birch, cajeput, laurel, or marjoram compress can also provide welcome relief when you suffer from sore muscles, muscle strain, or a stiff neck.

- Massage diluted juniper into stiff joints and muscles to relieve everyday aches and pains.

- Add a drop of lemon or orange to massage oils to help ease muscle pain.

- A hot bath with a drop of thyme or eucalyptus may soothe tired and aching muscles.

- To relieve muscle aches that accompany flu and fever, dilute five drops of palmarosa with a tablespoon of vegetable carrier oil and massage into the chest, shoulders, and neck.

- Massage the diluted oil of verbena into muscles to loosen them before a workout or to ease sore muscles afterward.

• Massage diluted Roman chamomile or lavender into affected areas to relieve muscle spasm.

NAUSEA

Nausea can be triggered by pregnancy, motion sickness, a migraine, or a virus. Sometimes it is simply a reaction to stress. The fragrance of the essential oil of peppermint can work in subtle physical and psychological ways to relieve nausea.

AROMATHERAPY FOR NAUSEA:

• Add a drop of peppermint oil to your bath.

• Rub your abdomen with a massage oil containing a drop of peppermint.

• Circulate the essential oil of peppermint through the air via an aroma lamp, ring, or diffuser.

• You may also disperse the scent of angelica through your environment to help combat nausea.

PMS

(*Premenstrual Syndrome*)

Many women experience both physical and emotional upset during the week before their period. Physical symptoms include water buildup, weight gain, and swollen, tender breasts, while emotional turmoil may take the form of irritability and mood swings. Supportive aromatherapy for PMS includes hot compresses, massages, and baths using essential oils.

AROMATHERAPY FOR PMS:

- To relieve the water buildup and irritability that often accompany PMS, use circular motions to massage the diluted essential oil of clary sage into the stomach and lower back. Roman chamomile or cardamom may also be helpful.

- Lavender is very calming and may be sniffed from a handkerchief, spritzed from a hydrolat, or diffused into the air to balance mood swings and promote stability. Clary sage and rose are also useful for this purpose.

- The scent of marjoram is very calming and may be diffused into the air, mixed with a massage oil or added to your bath to counteract the nervous tension associated with PMS.

- Add a few drops of juniper to your bath to help counteract the water buildup of PMS.

- A combination of ylang-ylang and lavender or clary sage in your bath may also help offset the mood swings of PMS.

- Lavender is very calming and may be inhaled to balance mood swings and promote stability.

- Try rubbing a massage oil containing basil in circles around the stomach area. The restorative qualities of basil oil may help regulate menstruation.

- Bergamot, neroli, or tangerine can be diffused into the air—or added to a bath, massage oil, or hot compress—to relieve premenstrual tension.

PRURITUS

Pruritus is the medical term for itching and can refer to intense itch on any area of the body. Frequently, however, it is used to refer to anal itch. Cool water and ice, frequent use of moisturizers, and oatmeal baths are steps you can take to control itching. If itching persists, see your doctor to determine if there is an underlying infection that requires treatment. Supportive aromatherapy for pruritus includes sitzbaths using essential oils.

AROMATHERAPY FOR PRURITUS:

• If you suffer from anal itch, prepare a warm sitzbath with one drop of lavender, tea tree, or rose in a bowl of warm water. Use once a day.

PSORIASIS

Psoriasis is a common skin problem characterized by circular patches of thickened red or pink skin. In conventional medicine steroids are prescribed to treat serious cases of psoriasis. Unfortunately steroids have a number of side effects.

Supportive aromatherapy for psoriasis includes the use of essential oils in massage oils, baths, and cool compresses. Dilute essential oils such as German chamomile and lavender with healing, anti-inflammatory carrier oils such as calendula and St. John's wort.

AROMATHERAPY FOR PSORIASIS:

• Combine several drops of German chamomile and lavender with a tablespoon of carrier oil such as calendula or St. John's wort. Apply to the affected areas via a massage oil, bath, or cool compress once or twice a day.

• Dilute three drops of birch, cade, cajeput, or everlasting with a tablespoon of a soothing carrier oil, and apply to the affected areas twice a day.

- Add a few drops of rosemary oil to your daily bath.

- Take a sponge bath using several drops of lemon or orange oil diluted with a quart of water.

- Apply a cool rose compress to affected areas.

SCARS

When a cut or wound heals, the blood clots over and seals it. Often there is a scab, and sometimes a scar results. Rubbing vitamin E into a scar and protecting the scar from sun exposure will help minimize its appearance. Supportive aromatherapy for the healing of scars involves the application of diluted essential oils.

AROMATHERAPY FOR SCARS:

- To speed healing from minor surgery, add several drops of everlasting (which breaks down scar tissue and eases discoloration) and rosemary (which stimulates local circulation) to a tablespoon of the base oil arnica. Apply up to three times daily. (After surgery consult your medical professional to make sure this preparation is right for you.)

- Combine five drops of angelica with a tablespoon of carrier oil and apply three times a day. (Avoid exposure to the sun directly after use.)

SEXUALITY

Certain essential oils have stimulating qualities, which has given them a reputation as aphrodisiacs. Essential oils that may act as sexual stimulants include rosemary, cedar, celery, and clove. At other moments more lush and sensual essential oils are appropriate. These richer, more earthy scents include clary sage, jasmine, patchouli, rose, sandalwood, and ylang-ylang. Choose your mood and your essential oil.

AROMATHERAPY FOR SEXUALITY:

- One of the above-mentioned essential oils may be circulated through the air via an aroma lamp, ring, or diffuser to reduce stress, relieve fatigue, and enhance sexuality.

- Add a few drops of the above-mentioned essential oil of your choice to a long and leisurely aromatic bath, alone or with your partner. You can also use these essential oils in the hot tub or sauna.

- Exchange slow and erotic massages with your partner, using several drops of your favorite stimulating or sensual essential oil diluted with a tablespoon of vegetable carrier oil.

- There are times when it's more appropriate to slow down, and the aroma of marjoram may discourage sexual desire.

SHINGLES

Shingles, or herpes zoster, is a painful outbreak of blisters and sores on the skin of adults who experienced chicken pox earlier in life. The virus may be reactivated by weakening of the immune system as you age, or possibly by stress. Your doctor may prescribe antiviral medications for this painful condition.

Supportive aromatherapy for shingles includes the application of essential oils to relieve the pain and itch of skin sores. Apply at the first sign of an attack to help prevent the virus from replicating.

AROMATHERAPY FOR SHINGLES:

- Dilute several drops of geranium with a tablespoon of vegetable carrier oil and place directly on sores, or apply a cool geranium compress.

- To relieve the itching and discomfort of shingles, add a few drops of peppermint to a mild lotion and apply to the affected areas.

- Apply a mixture of eight drops of myrtle diluted with a tablespoon of vegetable carrier oil.

Sinusitis

Sinusitis often accompanies or follows other upper respiratory infections such as colds and flu, and pollutants in the air we breathe may also be a contributing factor. A runny nose, congestion, headache, and difficulty sleeping may well add up to a case of sinusitis. While a persistent or severe case of sinusitis requires a trip to your doctor, supportive aromatherapy includes massages, baths, and diffusions of essential oils.

AROMATHERAPY FOR SINUSITIS:

- *Eucalyptus globulus* or *Eucalyptus radiata,* which are natural expectorants, may be inhaled several times a day to improve sinus congestion. Add three drops to a quart of hot water, cover your head with a towel, and rest your face about twelve inches above the bowl or pot. Breathe deeply. A drop or two of thyme or everlasting may also be used for this purpose.

- At night place a bowl of hot water containing one drop of eucalyptus and three drops of benzoin on your night table. Roman chamomile and thyme are also useful and may be substituted for eucalyptus. The aroma should help you clear stuffy sinuses, heal swollen membranes, and get a good night's sleep.

- Massage the sinus area with a drop of eucalyptus diluted with a tablespoon of vegetable carrier oil. You may also massage the chest with this preparation several times a day.

- Circulate eucalyptus through the air via an aroma lamp, ring, or diffuser, or add a few drops to your bath to relieve congestion.

- Several drops of niaouli, cajeput, or frankincense diluted with a tablespoon of vegetable carrier oil may also ease breathing difficulties. Massage the chest with this preparation several times a day.

- Diffuse angelica, cajeput, frankincense, or niaouli into the air to relieve congestion.

- As you recover, diffuse the warm, stimulating, and restorative scents of bay, cinnamon, or clove into the air.

- Inhaling the steam of cypress oil may have an overall beneficial effect on the respiratory system.

SKIN CARE

You can think of your skin—and especially your face—as a reflection of your personal habits over the course of your lifetime. Positive lifestyle choices such as a balanced diet and regular exercise contribute to your overall health, control the level of stress in your life, and strengthen your immune system—achievements that are in turn mirrored in the glow and luster of healthy, clear skin.

If you indulge in a poor diet or if you smoke, your complexion will gradually grow pale and sallow. The American Academy of Dermatology also warns us that up to 80 percent of what we once considered normal aging is actually photoaging—premature skin damage such as wrinkling and spotting due to long-term exposure to the sun.

Fortunately there are many natural ways you can care for your skin through the years, and aromatherapy can play an important role in these techniques. The therapeutic values of essential oils applied directly to the skin (in diluted form) can be evident as quickly as twenty minutes after use.

AROMATHERAPY FOR NORMAL SKIN:

• Maintain skin wellness with hydrolats, or floral waters. You can spritz your face with gentle, refreshing hydrolats on a daily basis. Rosewater and lavender are many women's favorite hydrolats for evenly balanced skin.

AROMATHERAPY FOR OILY SKIN:

• Add a drop of neroli to a lavender or rosewater hydrolat and spray several times a day on oily skin.

• Create a toning or astringent face oil. Dilute five drops of rosemary, geranium, or juniper with one tablespoon of a base oil such as apricot kernel, hazelnut, or sweet almond. Spritz a lavender hydrolat onto a cotton pad, add three to four drops of the face oil, and gently use a clean pad to dab any excess oil off the face. (You may also use the face oil alone on the pad, sans hydrolat.) Some women use toners every day, but unless you have exceptionally oily skin, it's best to use them once or twice a week.

- Try on a green clay mask. Clay masks of every variety are available at health food stores or by mail order, and green is considered the clay of choice. Green clay has natural healing and antiseptic qualities. Add a drop of rosemary, lavender, juniper, or patchouli to your mask to remove excess oil, tighten skin, soothe inflammation, and loosen blackheads. While the directions may differ slightly from product to product, you should generally cover your face with the smooth paste of the mask (avoiding the eyes and mouth) and let rest for fifteen minutes. Gently rinse and finish by applying a face oil, dabbing the face free of excess oil afterward. Use once a week.

- Make your own facial steambath. Add three to five drops of an essential oil such as anti-inflammatory lavender or stimulating rosemary to a quart of hot water. Cover your head with a towel and rest your face about twelve inches above the pot. Make sure that the water is not too hot. (This method is best used on oily skin to prevent acne from developing. Do *not* use facial steambaths when skin is already badly broken out, since steam creates—and can spread—bacteria.

AROMATHERAPY FOR DRY SKIN:

- Many essential oils act as natural moisturizers to give new life to dry skin. Helpful choices include lavender, bergamot, German chamomile, fennel, geranium, palmarosa, patchouli, sandalwood, and vetiver. Create your own moisturizing face and body oil by diluting three to five drops of an essential oil with a table-spoon of vegetable carrier oil. Apply with clean cotton pads.

• You may also add a drop of one of these essential oils to your own mild lotion or cream. Use lotions during the day, and feel free to slather on creams at night.

AROMATHERAPY FOR SENSITIVE SKIN:

• Add a drop of German chamomile to a lavender or rosewater hydrolat and spray several times a day on sensitive skin.

Also see **Acne** and **Aging Skin.**

SORE THROAT

Sore throats are an indication of an underlying respiratory ailment, such as a cold, flu, or bronchitis. Supportive aromatherapy involves the use of essential oils to relieve sore throat pain.

AROMATHERAPY FOR SORE THROATS:

• Gargle with a drop of marjoram, rose, sandalwood, or thyme oil mixed in a cup of water.

• For nighttime relief, place a bowl of hot water containing one drop of eucalyptus and three drops of benzoin at your bedside.

- Inhaling the steam of cypress oil may have an overall beneficial effect on the respiratory system.

SPIDER VEINS

Spider veins are actually weakened or broken capillaries just beneath the surface of the skin. They may be caused by a circulatory problem, but more often than not are simply part of the aging process. Supportive aromatherapy for spider veins consists of compresses and massages using essential oils.

AROMATHERAPY FOR SPIDER VEINS:

- Calendula, carrot, cypress, neroli, palmarosa, parsley, and rose may all be helpful treatments for spider veins.

- Apply a cool compress made with one or more of these essential oils once a day.

- Massage affected areas with several drops of one or more of these essential oils diluted with a tablespoon of vegetable carrier oil. Apply once a day at bedtime.

STOMACHACHE

A stomachache is an indication of digestive problems. Perhaps you have a poor diet, don't get enough exercise, or find yourself under a great deal of stress. If stomachaches become chronic, you should see your doctor to rule out any serious underlying health problems. Supportive aromatherapy for stomachaches includes hot compresses, massages, and diffusions of essential oils.

AROMATHERAPY FOR STOMACHACHES:

- Place a hot Roman-chamomile or cajeput compress on your stomach. Roman chamomile is especially useful in treating the tummy troubles of children, since it is soothing yet extremely mild.

- Massage your stomach area with several drops of the essential oils of angelica, cajeput, chamomile, fennel, or rosemary diluted with a tablespoon of vegetable carrier oil. Fennel is especially useful in this regard.

- Diffuse the essential oil of peppermint into the air to help relieve a stomachache accompanied by nausea.

STRESS

Stress consists of anxiety and tension, usually in response to events in your day-to-day life. Serious events, such as the loss of a loved one, a job change, or a move can create acute stress. Others of us live in a chronic state of stress due to a difficult marriage or career or financial difficulties.

Stress is a serious problem. Besides the unpleasant sensation in and of itself, stress can lead to health problems such as depression, high blood pressure, and a lowered immune system. While the ideal solution is to eliminate the underlying cause of stress, aromatherapy offers supportive strategies. Many essential oils may help you combat stress. Experiment with different essential oils until you find the one that is right for you. Over time you may find that you enjoy combining oils for a synergistic effect.

AROMATHERAPY FOR STRESS:

- The essential oils of Roman chamomile, clary sage, everlasting, fennel, frankincense, geranium, lavender, marjoram, melissa, neroli, orange, rose, sandalwood, tangerine, vanilla, vetiver, and ylang-ylang are all renowned for their abilities to counteract the effects of daily stress.

- Dilute several drops of a calming essential oil with a tablespoon of vegetable carrier oil or mild lotion and massage into the body. A full-body massage is one of the most effective ways to alleviate symptoms brought on by stress. Not only does this process encourage relaxation, it actually causes your body to release endorphins, which are natural painkillers and increase your sense of pleasure. Any of the essential oils mentioned above are perfect for a massage blend.

• Diffuse one or more of these oils into the environment to release tension and anxiety.

• Create a soothing aromatic experience by adding a few drops of one of these essential oils to your regular bath.

SUNBURN

While a serious sunburn requires medical attention, minor sunburns respond well to home treatment with aromatherapy. (The wisest course to follow is to use plenty of sunscreen and protect yourself from getting a sunburn in the first place.)

AROMATHERAPY FOR SUNBURN:

• Apply cold lavender compresses to affected areas. A combination of lavender and aloe vera can be particularly helpful in this case.

TOOTHACHE

Serious toothaches require a trip to the dentist. In the meantime supportive aromatherapy for toothaches consists mainly of pain relief with the local application of essential oils.

AROMATHERAPY FOR TOOTHACHES:

• To relieve the pain of a toothache, place a drop of peppermint oil on a sterile cotton swab and press gently against the affected area.

• Use a drop of diluted clove oil on a cotton swab to numb pain. A brief application (less than a minute) should be sufficient. Longer use may lead to local irritation.

• Gargle with a mouthwash containing myrrh, or make your own mouthwash by adding a drop of myrrh to a cup of water. (Do not swallow.)

• A special note on babies: Very few remedies are gentle enough for very young children. Roman chamomile is an exception. To relieve baby's teething pain, dilute a drop of the essential oil of chamomile with a tablespoon of vegetable carrier oil and rub a small amount directly on the gums.

URINARY TRACT INFECTIONS

Annoying, inconvenient, and sometimes quite painful, urinary tract infections are much more common in women than in men. They are characterized by burning upon urination and a frequent need to urinate. If urinary tract infections become chronic, you should see your doctor to rule out any serious underlying health problems. Supportive aromatherapy for urinary tract infections includes baths, sitzbaths, and massages using essential oils.

AROMATHERAPY FOR URINARY TRACT INFECTIONS:

- Add a few drops of lavender oil to a sitzbath and use after urination.

- Add a drop or two of bergamot to a sitzbath. Use once a day.

- Add a few drops of juniper oil to a sitzbath. Use once a day. (Do *not* use for kidney infections.)

- Use gentle circular motions to rub a massage oil containing niaouli, cajeput, or sandalwood into the abdomen and kidney region in the lower back. (Niaouli is traditionally considered most effective for this purpose.)

- Add a few drops of essential pine oil to the bath, or massage the diluted oil of pine in circles around the abdomen.

VAGINITIS

Vaginitis occurs when the vagina becomes inflamed due to infection with yeast, bacteria, or protozoa, taking certain medications (such as antibiotics or birth control pills), wearing tight pants, tampon use, obesity, or diabetes. The discharge, itching, and occasionally foul odor of vaginitis can be both uncomfortable and embarrassing. A case of vaginitis often requires a trip (or at least a phone call) to your gynecologist. Supportive aromatherapy for vaginitis consists of sitzbaths and massages.

AROMATHERAPY FOR VAGINITIS:

- One of the most promising new treatments for vaginitis is tea tree oil. Both French and American studies have shown that tea tree has enormous potential in treating vaginal yeast infections. Try it in a sitzbath or dilute with a tablespoon of vegetable carrier oil and apply to the affected area twice a day.

- Add several drops of lavender or juniper oil to a sitzbath and use once a day.

- Take a yarrow sitzbath once a day. To make, dilute three drops of yarrow oil with two cups of rosewater.

- Add a few drops of essential pine oil to your bath, or massage the diluted oil in circles around the stomach area.

VARICOSE VEINS

Swollen, purple varicose veins occur when circulation from your heart is constricted by weight gain, constipation, or pregnancy. Usually they appear on your legs; varicose veins in the rectal area are hemorrhoids. To cope with varicose veins, try to keep your feet elevated, exercise, and avoid remaining on your feet for prolonged periods of time. Massaging essential oils into the legs once a day may increase circulation and help reduce the swelling or prevent the development of varicose veins.

AROMATHERAPY FOR VARICOSE VEINS:

- Dilute several drops of everlasting with a tablespoon of vegetable carrier oil and gently massage over your varicose veins. Do not apply pressure to the affected veins. The essential oils of calendula, cypress, juniper, lavender, rosemary, and yarrow may also be helpful.

- Add a few drops of these essential oils to your bath or shower. If you like, pour a few drops onto a sponge or washcloth and lightly massage over varicose veins, lather and rinse.

WOUNDS

Many cuts and scrapes can be cleaned and disinfected with your own natural first-aid kit. Essential oils such as lavender, tea tree, calendula, eucalyptus, lemon, and thyme have antiseptic and healing properties. Any serious wound of course requires medical attention.

AROMATHERAPY FOR WOUNDS:

- The best remedies for wounds are lavender and tea tree. Apply a drop of the neat (undiluted) essential oil directly to the cut or scrape to promote healing.

- Combine five drops of angelica with a tablespoon of carrier oil and apply three times a day. (Avoid exposure to the sun directly after use.)

- Apply a hot calendula compress to a wound to stop bleeding and promote healing.

- A drop or two of eucalyptus may be applied to cleanse minor cuts and scrapes.

- Combine a drop of lemon with a teaspoon of the carrier oil arnica to clean cuts and wounds and stop them from bleeding.

- A drop of thyme oil added to a mild lotion may be used to disinfect minor cuts and scrapes.

FOR MORE INFORMATION

FURTHER READING

Complete Aromatherapy Handbook, by Susanne Fischer-Rizzi, Sterling Publishing Co., 1990.

Aromatherapy, by Daniele Ryman, Bantam Books, 1993.

Aromatherapy for Women, by Maggie Tisserand, Healing Arts Press, 1988.

The Art of Aromatherapy, by Robert B. Tisserand, Destiny Books, 1989.

The Complete Book of Essential Oils and Aromatherapy, by Valerie Ann Worwood, New World Library, 1991.

USEFUL ADDRESSES

American Aromatherapy Association
P.O. Box 1222
Fair Oaks, CA 95628

Aromatherapy and Herbal Studies
219 Carl Street
San Francisco, CA 94117
Phone: (415) 564-6785
Fax: (415) 564-6799

Aromatherapy Seminars
3379 Robertson Boulevard
Los Angeles, CA 90034
Phone: (310) 838-6122

B.C. Botanicus
Red Horse Complex, Unit #1
74 Montauk Highway
East Hampton, NY 11937
Phone: (516) 329-2525
        (800) 669-7618
Fax: (516) 329-2196

Institute of Classical Aromatherapy
P.O. Box 98
936 Peace Portal Drive
Blaine, WA 98231
Phone: (800) 260-7401

Leydet Aromatics
P.O. Box 2354
Fair Oaks, CA 95628
Phone: (916) 965-7546
Fax: (916) 962-3292

Lotus Light
P.O. Box 1008
Wilmot, WI 53170
Phone: (414) 889-8501

National Association for Holistic Aromatherapy
P.O. Box 17622
Boulder, CO 80308
Phone: (303) 258-3791

Original Swiss Aromatics
P.O. Box 6842
602 Freitas Parkway
San Rafael, CA 94903
Phone: (415) 459-3998
Fax: (415) 479-0614

The Pacific Institute of Aromatherapy
P.O. Box 6723
San Rafael, CA 94903
Phone: (415) 479-9121
Fax: (415) 479-0614

*

INDEX